Navigate Your Beauty

Smart and Safe Plastic Surgery Solutions

Rod J. Rohrich, M.D.
Mary Crosland

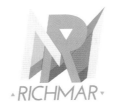

Contents

Acknowledgments

This book is written for the consumer and has required a considerable, combined effort from all those who have been heavily associated with this endeavor. These individuals have made this experience a truly worthwhile and positive one.

We thank Diane Sinn, my tireless senior administrator, who has been with me for over twenty-five years, for her focus, effort, editing, and common-sense approach. We also thank Patricia Aitson, my long-time, superb photographer, who helped us with all the great photographs, and Martha Aceves for her creative ability as a fabulous illustrator. We also thank Steven Connell, our webmaster, for his talent in ramping up our website. We thank Julie Meyer, Amy Ryan, and Alice Sutherland, assistants to Mary Crosland, for their excellent editing and organization, and for keeping us focused and going forward to get it done. We are grateful to Michael Levin and Sara Stratton for their editorial expertise. We give our utmost thanks to James W. Dunn for his superb creative and design capabilities.

We are very appreciative and express our gratitude to the *Journal of Plastic and Reconstructive Surgery* for giving us permission to use selected patient photographs from articles published by Dr. Rohrich for our book.

Last, but not least, we would like to thank all the patients who gave their priceless and invaluable input. Their personal experiences, questions, and comments are what gave us the true insight to write this book to provide safety for all consumers.

Preface
The Three Magic Questions

Beauty is a lifelong journey.

We're here to help you navigate that journey, so you can discover the facts about plastic surgery for yourself. What are the key procedures you should consider? What's the right age for each option? What can you expect, during your surgery, immediately afterward, and in the months and years to come?

The single most important decision you'll make as you navigate your beauty is *choosing the right surgeon.* We'll show you exactly how to do just that.

It's so easy to choose the wrong one as many advertise to do plastic surgery, but are not even plastic surgeons. You see them on billboards, in city magazines, even on late night TV ads, offering discounts, cut-rate surgeries, and promises that are simply too good to be true. And yet, people fall into their hands every day, sometimes with disastrous consequences.

You can have safe and successful plastic surgery if you know how to find the right practitioners, and this book will show you how to identify them, interview them, and work with them to create the best possible outcome for your appearance and self-image.

It will take a little bit of effort for you to find the best, but that effort will be repaid many times over, in the way you look and feel about yourself.

Those who don't make that effort can pay a terrible price, not just in financial terms but also in their appearance, their self-image, and possibly their health.

We are here to make sure this doesn't happen to you!

This book is packed with real-world guidance from one of America's top plastic surgeons and a patient who is a Dallas businesswoman, very savvy consumer, and a thorough studier of plastic surgery.

But our most important gift, indeed the foundation of this book, is a method for identifying the right plastic surgeon for you ... no matter where you live, no matter what procedure you contemplate.

WE CALL OUR METHOD THE *THREE MAGIC QUESTIONS*.

These questions will help you narrow down your choices to the best and safest practitioners. Photocopy the *Three Magic Questions* or even tear them out of the book, and keep them with you. Make them the foundation of your research as you begin the process to navigate your beauty! If you don't get satisfying answers to these three questions, move on. Your appearance and your health are far too vital to leave in the hands of amateurs.

In his best-selling book, *Outliers*, Malcolm Gladwell writes that in any given field it takes 10,000 hours of experience to reach expert status. Has the surgeon you're considering put in those 10,000 hours or more? Most board certified plastic surgeons have done so by the time they complete all their training and certification by the American Board of Plastic Surgery. If not, do you want to be the surgical equivalent of a practice round? We doubt it. You must choose a highly experienced plastic surgeon—someone who's already at the top of his or her field and not someone on the way up or down. Let them get their experience with someone other than you! This is where the *Three Magic Questions* will not fail you—experts see and do things that others never do!

We think these questions are magical because they reveal in an instant whether you are dealing with a trustworthy professional or someone who could do you far more harm than good. They also level the playing field in an instant. Normally, when patients meet practitioners, the spacious, attractive offices, the white lab coat on the doctor, and the diplomas on the wall (some of which may mean absolutely nothing!) can awe them. Patients often don't know what to ask or are afraid to ask anything at all, because they're concerned they'll offend the doctor. Remember that he or she is there to serve you, not the other way around. When you ask these three questions, it really is like magic. The fancy surroundings no longer matter. You are quickly cutting to the heart of the matter—is this individual qualified to perform a given type of plastic surgery on you safely and with a high probability of a good outcome?

Here are the *Three Magic Questions* to ask any plastic surgeon* into whose hands you are entrusting your beauty and your health:

1. **Is this one of the top three surgeries you perform and how often do you do it?** Choose a surgeon for whom this procedure is one of their top three, with a minimum of at least one of these procedures per week over the past five years. Now you know he or she has the **Experience** you demand for the procedure you want.

2. **Do you teach, speak, or write about this procedure for the benefit of other plastic surgeons?** The answer will quickly reveal the surgeon's level of **Expertise** and respect by his peers in the procedure you desire.

3. **Do you have long-term follow-up photos for this procedure?** As the prospective patient, you should like the results you see. Insist on seeing/reviewing at least two or more long-term (more than one year) patient results for the procedure you are considering. You need to see consistent, **Exceptional results** you really like.

Simply put, your surgeon must have the **Experience, Expertise,** and show **Exceptional results**. The Three E's.

Keep these *Three Magic Questions* in mind as you read this book and go on the exciting journey to navigate your beauty!

Rod J. Rohrich, M.D.
Mary Crosland

* Certified by the American Board of Plastic Surgery (ABPS)

So You're Considering Plastic Surgery!

We'll start with the good news: For most people, plastic surgery can safely create a more beautiful you. In the hands of an accomplished plastic surgeon, you can literally turn back the hands of time. Procedures exist to improve virtually every aspect of your appearance. Not everyone is a candidate for plastic surgery, and not everyone who claims to be a plastic surgeon is trained to do these delicate and complex procedures. This book will show you how to match your needs and desires for a more attractive you with the right procedures. **Even more importantly, we'll show you how to find the best trained, most qualified, and compassionate plastic surgeon for whatever procedure you choose.**

In short, we will show you how to *navigate your beauty*.

If this book serves no other purpose, it will keep you out of the hands of unqualified practitioners.

As you'll discover, any doctor can call himself a plastic surgeon, even with little more than a weekend's worth of training in the field. Every day, there are patients who subject themselves to surgery in the hands of individuals who aren't even doctors! Consumers are woefully uninformed and put themselves, their appearance, and their health at considerable risk.

Let me share with you a story of plastic surgery gone wrong, so you can see exactly what I want to help you avoid.

When Julie came to see me the first time, she was in tears as she had had four rhinoplasty procedures (nose jobs) over the course of the previous two years. Her nose was entirely collapsed, scarred, and had a depressed dimple on her nasal tip. I explained to her that she would have to wait a year to fully heal before I could attempt revision surgery to undo some of the damage. I also explained that she would need a rib graft to reconstruct her nose. To add insult to injury, she had just found out that her "cosmetic surgeon" was not a plastic surgeon or an oto-laryngologist (ENT—ear, nose, and throat doctor)—both of these surgeons are qualified to perform rhinoplasty. He was a dentist without a license to perform surgery.

Stories like this happen more than they should, but it doesn't have to be this way. Fortunately, for this patient, the new results were positive and she now looks great and can once again breathe through her nose.

This is one of the reasons I am writing this book. This is for you, as a consumer, to become your best advocate, to educate yourself, and to find the best plastic surgeon for you—a true expert who cares about you! Most people spend more time finding a pair of shoes than researching who will do their plastic surgery.

You don't want to fall into the wrong doctor's hands—someone who has had no more than a weekend's worth of training and is now performing plastic surgery just because he or she can do it at their office. Yes, right here in the United States, a physician can do this. It is truly frightening what you can do once you get your M.D. license—you can call yourself whatever you like. **Plastic surgery has become a "buyer-beware" specialty.** For example, you will see people working in a spa with no medical training at all injecting substances into their clients' faces. It could be a real filler or not—who knows.

There are doctors who advertise on billboards who are not surgeons, let alone real plastic surgeons. Doctors may also offer cut-rate surgery to large numbers of patients with little to no regard for the health and well-being of the people ostensibly under their care. They may never see their patients pre- or post-op. This is a well-kept deception in medicine that is occurring every day in every major city in this nation.

My co-author, Mary Crosland, and I are going to help you avoid this from happening. Read this book and arm yourself with the knowledge to select the best, real plastic surgeon.

Unfortunately, these are real life nightmares that I see almost daily in my practice. In the media, these cases are often referred to as "plastic surgery gone wrong." But it is not even plastic surgery in most cases, since it was not even done by a plastic surgeon. I've seen so many of these patients, in my waking life and, without exaggeration, in my nightmares, too. I feel it is time to speak out and help you as a consumer to be wise and informed. I am a board certified plastic surgeon who specializes in cosmetic and revision surgery, among other things, and am professor and chairman of the Department of Plastic Surgery at the University of Texas Southwestern Medical Center in Dallas, Texas. I have my private practice at the Dallas Plastic Surgery Institute.

With so many guides already written on plastic surgery, you may be wondering why the world could possibly need another. **I saw a need for a guide that focuses on giving you the tools to take charge of your own health and to navigate your life and your beauty, while putting special emphasis on safety.** I wanted to create a comprehensive guide to all things plastic surgery, ranging from basic skin care to safe plastic surgery solutions. I hope you will find this book useful regardless of your age or aesthetic needs.

Although I have frequently expressed these concerns at conferences with my colleagues, the time has come to explain to consumers what plastic surgery is and how to navigate safe and positive outcomes. Julie, and patients like her, became my tipping point in writing this book for you. After seeing so many patients over the years that have had a deep-seated need to understand the facts related to plastic surgery procedures, I knew I had to write this book, *Navigate Your Beauty: Smart and Safe Plastic Surgery Solutions.*

This guide will help you find your way to the best care in all of plastic surgery and beyond. We will give you the basics of how to find the best skin care, how to find the best plastic surgeon, how to know what you may need done and when to do it. We will help you reach smart and safe decisions!

This topic has been a lifelong personal crusade for me. I have wanted to write this book for over twenty years, though I could not do so until I found the right partner. I wanted to provide not only the expertise and knowledge of a surgeon, but also the perspective and insight of a knowledgeable and savvy patient/consumer. Without the right co-author with that insight and intellect to get the job done correctly, I could not go forward with the project. Fortunately, I have now found that person in my co-author, Mary Crosland. Mary is a beautiful and successful businesswoman, and more importantly, a savvy consumer who understands from all angles, pre-op to post-op to recovery with several friends, and has gone through the plastic surgery process herself.

Together, Mary and I will provide the two essential points of view: that of an experienced surgeon and that of a well-informed patient/consumer. With my surgical expertise and her first-person insight into being a diligent patient and a smart consumer, we will describe the plastic surgery process in a way that eliminates the unknown and, we hope, removes your own apprehensions. We know that this may be one of the most exciting decisions you will make, and are proud to assist you in the process of what we call "navigating your beauty." Together, we hope to educate and empower you so you can take charge of your own health and beauty.

If you are considering plastic surgery, you need all of the facts so you can weigh your options and proceed cautiously, yet confidently. Your surgery should be a physically and emotionally life-enhancing event that will leave you looking and feeling your best. So take the time to prepare yourself—this book is the perfect place to start. **We will educate you about the entire field of cosmetic plastic surgery, focusing not only on results, but also on the full process leading up to and following your surgery. Your appearance is your unique and special identity, and is a major part of who you are as an individual.**

Every surgery, even a seemingly minor or routine one, carries the reality of risks. Any time you are feeling strained or anxious about your research, we hope you will pause. Your journey must be made with internal conviction and be guided by truth, not a sales pitch or an idealized body you see in the media. Take your time, read the whole book, or at least all of the chapters relevant to the procedure(s) you are considering, and you will find yourself able to navigate that journey and enhance your own beauty.

First and foremost, we want to help you find the right surgeon for your procedure so you don't become another statistic. There's no need for this! Plastic surgery, when performed by a qualified expert, is very safe and very effective.

You may be wondering who I am. My name is Rod J. Rohrich. I am a husband (married to Diane L. Gibby—also a board certified plastic surgeon), father of two, and an internationally recognized plastic surgeon as well as a global leader in the field. I am board certified by the American Board of Plastic Surgery and am known for my passion and compassion in patient care. I am also a professor and the chairman of the Department of Plastic Surgery at the University of Texas Southwestern Medical Center. I believe in total patient care and am committed to each of my patients, not just in the short term, but also for the rest of their lives! I serve patients of all ages, from those in their early teens to mature adults. **Above all, I recognize that there is a story behind each patient, and that every procedure is part of a larger doctor–patient relationship.**

My involvement in the field includes innovatively researching the development of new cosmetic treatments, teaching the next generation of plastic surgery experts, and operating on patients five days a week. I have been fully trained in all aspects of plastic surgery. My private practice and university practice span all conceivable treatments, from fillers to breast augmentation to rhinoplasty to facelifts, as well as body contouring and complex reconstructive surgery. My education includes a total of fifteen years of training—four in undergrad, four in medical school, six specializing in plastic surgery, and one final year of fellowship training. I have spent my career and my life perfecting my art to provide the best care for my patients. My training and learning is ongoing (as it should be for any medical practitioner).

Do I Need Plastic Surgery?

Most people considering plastic surgery fall into one of two camps. The first is comprised of people who are happy with their appearance, but still find themselves wondering—*what if?* The other group knows they want help and usually arrives at my office with a detailed work list. These two camps are not that far apart in their thinking. If you are still in the wondering phase, my goal is to help educate you to find what you really want. This book will arm you with the material you need to confront your curiosities or reservations. My goal is to instill a sense of confidence in you, so you can trust yourself to make the right decision. You are making very special and important decisions here that are unlike any other large consumer choices you will likely make. This is bigger than buying a house or a new car—this is *YOU.*

The origin of the word "plastic" in plastic surgery comes from a Greek derivation meaning "the means to mold or to make." So this is the ultimate "makeover," the ultimate lifestyle choice, and it is individualized to you. Plastic surgery is not a generic, one-size-fits-all service, despite what some practitioners may believe.

Here's an exercise for you to begin with—what we call the Mirror Test. Look in the mirror and list the three things you most want to change about your appearance. Be honest and practical. Decide whether or not the time is right for you and whether or not you are ready to make the enhancement. Bottom line—will these changes help you be a better version of yourself?

If you've already been to a surgeon's office, chances are you have a good idea of what you would like to change. The choice of surgeon will be your first and most important decision as a consumer and patient. I want this book to empower you to find the right plastic surgeon for you and your procedure.

Genetically, everyone ages differently and everyone will recover from surgery differently. A facelift at forty-five or fifty will look better than a facelift at sixty-five or seventy. Regardless of age, you want to look as good as possible—today and ten years from now. **Remember, *looking good* goes hand in hand with *feeling good.*** This is one of the miracles of plastic surgery: the psychological manifestations of a fresher exterior. So, do you want plastic surgery? Ask yourself—could you look and feel better? After reading this book and becoming informed about the options available to you, you can identify how a procedure can achieve your specific goals.

Surgery is not always the answer. Have you ever seen those pictures of the "Cat Woman"? I'm not talking about the character from *Batman*, but the woman who is often featured in tabloid magazines in the grocery aisles. She has had a lot of so-called "plastic surgery." She has had so much work done that she no longer looks like herself ... or even like a human being!

This is definitely *not* the kind of plastic surgery that I practice, nor is it the type of plastic surgery practiced by most of the board certified plastic surgeons in the United States. **A plastic surgeon is a physician first and foremost, and *then* a plastic surgeon, upholding the highest ethical standards.** I live and work by the Hippocratic Oath, which means I've sworn not to do you harm, and this is the foundation of what you want from your chosen surgeon. The last thing you need is a consultation with a plastic surgeon willing to turn you into somebody looking like a "Cat Woman" for a price. A true, ethical surgeon acts with consideration for the true needs of the patient. He or she will enrich your humanity, not erase it. Part of navigating your beauty is navigating the system of finding the right board certified plastic surgeon for you. We will show you how to get the very best surgeon and how to do it easily.

Anxiety over looking like "Cat Woman" is an extreme manifestation of a common concern among my patients. Prospective patients are often afraid that surgery will leave them looking like someone else. Perhaps they have friends who had surgery and no longer look like themselves. No one wants this. The purpose of a procedure is to improve and enhance your beauty, not to change yourself into someone else. This may be the case if you are not careful to select the proper surgeon. **I like to say that we are in the face protection, not witness protection, program!** We want to make you look and feel good, and I am not willing to make you look like somebody else.

Beautiful women often come into my office and want me to operate on them. Even though they look great, they want to look *better*. The procedures I perform correct problems these women don't suffer from, and they would see no results. **An honest plastic surgeon has to be able to say NO if the patient does not need or is not ready, physically or emotionally, for a given cosmetic procedure.** I encounter this often in my clinical practice, such as a patient who wants more lip filler when she does not need it. If I were to do more lip fillers in such a situation, she would look unnatural and almost sour. It is not normal for your upper lip to look bigger than your lower lip. My sense of ethics, as well as my sense of beauty and aesthetic harmony, prevent me from ever doing such a procedure—and you should never allow anyone to do such a number on you!

This is why choosing the right surgeon is so important. Do your due diligence and be sure he or she is a true expert in the procedure you are considering. You want a surgeon who listens to every question you have and has the expertise and intuition to hear the real concerns *behind* the questions. Every aspect of your procedure should be explained in such reassuring detail that you leave the office without a lingering doubt. Your surgeon must be approachable, concerned, authoritative, and have patience with your concerns. Don't be swayed by a white coat or credentials of unknown legitimacy hung on the wall. **Don't be swayed by a great website—everyone is famous on their own website.** If you are not personally comfortable with the individual, you should move on and consider another surgeon to handle your care.

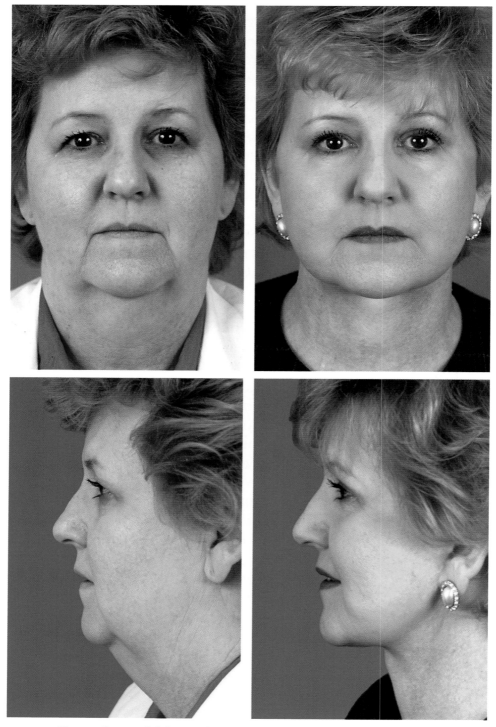

Natural, youthful result with modern "Lift and Fill" facial rejuvenation

The right practitioner will pass the Three A's with flying colors. He or she should be Amiable, Available, and of course, Able. But just as important are the Three C's—they should be Caring, Compassionate, and Completely empathetic to you and your needs!

We will go deeper into the process of selecting the right surgeon in Chapter 3. For now, just understand that it is the first and most important decision you will make as a patient and consumer.

Now I want to introduce you to my wonderful co-author, Mary Crosland. Throughout this book, Mary's comments will always be in italics so you know who's speaking at any given time.

My name is Mary Crosland. I am a wife, a mother, a successful business owner, and have been a patient of Dr. Rohrich for years. For the last four years, I have owned and operated a salon in Dallas. In the salon world, as in the field of plastic surgery, we understand how important physical appearance is to your overall well-being. To succeed in both of these businesses, you have to understand and appreciate beauty and aesthetics as well as business, professional consistency, and customer satisfaction. This is one of the reasons I admire Dr. Rohrich so much—he also serves the needs of a demanding clientele, and he does so with incredible experience, expertise, knowledge, and a true compassion for his "clients."

As someone who is also in the business of making people look more beautiful, I believe that there is a certain magic, if you will, to plastic surgery. It can enhance our natural physical beauty and assist in the efforts we make to take care of ourselves. Dr. Rohrich is, in my opinion, a master not just with a scalpel but also with his vision. He sees not only the individual in his office for a consultation, but also the person his patients want to be after surgery and recovery. He is an artist in the surgical studio in the same manner as Degas or Renoir. You will be very glad you got to know him through this book.

During our emergency room visit in the middle of the night, a deep friendship and trust between the two of us was born and has only solidified over time. While the conditions under which we met were unfortunate, I am nonetheless thankful that we did meet and get to know one another. This is why I wanted to do this book with him—to help others find the kind of surgeon and physician that I have found.

I had been hospitalized following a complication from a procedure. I would never have expected one of the world's leading plastic surgeons to come to the hospital at four in the morning to aid a patient he had only recently met. His patient care, compassion, and expertise are beyond reproach.

Many of my friends come to me for direction when they begin to consider a cosmetic procedure or plastic surgery. I have experienced it myself and have also done plenty of personal research. These same friends ask me questions about the various procedures available to them—what to expect during surgery and then in recovery, even what to pack for their trip to the hospital! Recently, a friend of mine said to me, "Okay, if someone would've shown me a picture of what I was going to look like on day seven or eight of my recovery after my laser peel, I would not have been so freaked out when I saw it!" I knew exactly what she meant. It was all very normal how she looked, but she would have been better prepared on what each day would bring and had far less worries. I also knew that on or about day fourteen, she was going to look great, and she did.

A light bulb went off in my head! We can show people what to expect so they don't have as much anxiety during the process. This is why I co-wrote this book with Dr. Rohrich—to provide others with the same kind of guidance I provide for all my friends and acquaintances, and the guidance he has provided me.

Dr. Rohrich and I felt that the beauty and uniqueness of this book would be its dual perspectives, his and mine, doctor and patient/consumer. I know that, together, we can provide valuable resources for potential patients—what to expect, what to plan, how the whole process works— answering questions, easing concerns, and calming fears!

Dr. Rohrich has written hundreds of medical articles and many textbooks on plastic surgery, and is a leader in his field worldwide. These textbooks, however, are written to teach other surgeons the art and advances in plastic surgery. With this unique book, we seek to provide the missing link with a comprehensive guide to the ins and outs of plastic surgery with the patient in mind. Most likely, you didn't go to medical school—neither did I. But I do know the actual steps of the plastic surgery process—facts, feelings, and even finances. This is the unique view I bring.

In this way, the book is a perfect triangle. One point is the professional doctor, another is the satisfied patient, and the third is you.

I want to stress that even with this book, you will need to set up a support system. The post-operative process, or post-op for short, can be very trying for both men and women. For example, some anxiety and depression are common. **To have someone there is very important and why I advise you to have a surgery companion to help you through the process. I do this for my friends who are patients of Dr. Rohrich. They had <u>me</u>. Now, through this book, you've got a "me" as well!**

Everyone needs a Mary (your surgical companion)—someone who understands and can guide and walk with them through pre- and post-op care and recovery. This makes such an important difference, so enjoy the book, keep it at your bedside for reference, and take it with you when you visit your plastic surgeon. They will take notice that you are being proactive about your own care and life.

Mary is right: You should work on building your real support network as well as finding a great surgeon. Your support network needs to be those you can trust and depend on to learn about your procedure with you, and to be there when you need them.

While you build up your own personal support and medical network, consider Mary and myself your greatest resources and your first-line authorities. We really want the very best for you. It is better to pay more for a true professional and get your procedure done right the first time, than go through the nightmare of multiple revision surgeries to correct mistakes.

A relationship with a plastic surgeon is usually not a one off event. Ideally, it develops into a long-term partnership where you and your plastic surgeon work together to determine what is needed to look your best at any given age and stage of life.

In the next chapter, we'll discuss what is appropriate in each decade of life and how plastic surgery can be a lifelong benefit to you and those you love.

Five Key Points to Remember:

1. This book will give you guidance from both the consumer and plastic surgeon perspective.

2. Know what you would like to improve or enhance—take the Mirror Test.

3. Understand that plastic surgery is generally safe and effective—but only when performed properly.

4. Picking the correct plastic surgeon is your first and most important task. Seek the best in a surgeon—someone with the Three C's and the Three A's.

5. A supportive "surgery companion" to accompany you through the process is essential to round out your support network.

What and When—
Because It's All About You!

2

Navigating your beauty is a lifelong journey. With an outstanding plastic surgeon as your partner and guide, you can enhance different aspects of your appearance as the years go by. So here's a question we'll address in this chapter: What procedures and surgical options are appropriate in each decade of your life?

Some solutions discussed here are surgical and others are not, so you'll need a surgeon who understands both **aesthetic surgery** and **cosmetic medicine** to ensure you are getting the right care. That surgeon can also help you build a network of physicians in different specialties as you need them. **Here is a secret of medicine:** *Great physicians will refer you to other great physicians.* **There are doctors and then there are world-class doctors**. We'll show you how to find the best of the best, but for now, let's examine what a lifelong journey of enhancing your beauty entails.

Teens (and Younger Children)

Teenagers rarely need to correct wrinkles, sagging skin, or anything else caused by age, sun, and gravity. However, young people with physical differences, such as large noses, protruding ears, or skin disorders may feel self-conscious about these issues. Plastic surgery can shape the nose or reset the ears. Minimally invasive treatments such as laser hair removal and medical skin care can help remove unwanted hair and embarrassing skin conditions, such as early onset acne.

What is an appropriate age for a child or teenager to have plastic surgery? It depends upon the patient. Corrective ear surgery can be done as early as age six and nose reshaping as early as age fifteen in females and seventeen in males. Female breast reduction can be done between the ages of fifteen and seventeen, or once the breasts are fully developed. Treatment for gynecomastia correction (male breast reduction—this can be present in up to 20 percent of all males) can also be done between the age of fifteen and seventeen.

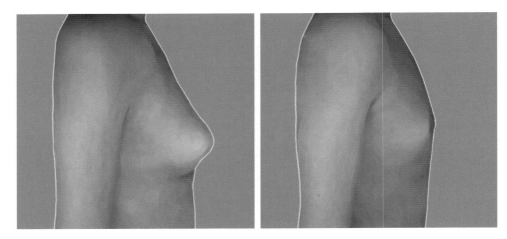

Illustration of male breast reduction (gynecomastia) using ultrasound liposuction only

These are the most commonly performed surgeries in teens. Non-operative, non-invasive techniques include microdermabrasion for skin toning and refreshing, unwanted hair elimination using laser hair removal, and good medical-grade skin care to help correct or improve acne. These are generally safe to perform at an earlier age—speak with your surgeon about your child's situation.

The media often portrays teenagers getting plastic surgery as inappropriate. If it's just about enhancing appearance, I agree. But teens who have one of the corrective procedures Dr. Rohrich just mentioned often experience amazing boosts in self-confidence. Afterward, they often perform better in school and especially in social activities, all of which are stressful enough without having to struggle with the continued worry about physical appearance and normalcy. It can be a confidence builder.

I have observed remarkable transformations in young girls and boys after they undergo simple corrective procedures, such as fixing bat ears or a prominent nose. These are often sources of humiliation—kids, as we know, can be cruel (especially to each other)—and giving these children their self-confidence back is one of the most rewarding things I do. During follow-up appointments, I commonly see an evolution in personality. A simple ear alteration can change the attitude of a young girl or boy for the remainder of his or her life.

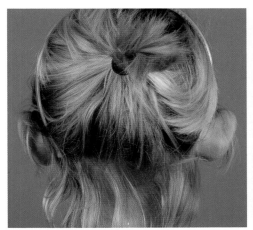 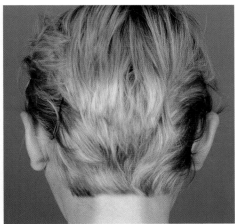

Correction of prominent ears in a 10-year-old boy

The goal is not to convince teens that they need to change but rather to help them gain control of the areas that are causing them unhappiness or embarrassment. Teens are very sensitive, impressionable, and vulnerable, and I well understand the need to be careful when guiding younger patients. We can make someone look better on the outside, but this may not always transfer to the inside unless the patient is ready and willing to do so. For example, I saw a fourteen-year-old young girl who was forty pounds overweight for her age and height. She did not need liposuction. Rather, she needed counseling and nutritional care to restore and rebuild her body image and self-esteem. I referred her to a life coach, who helped her alter her lifestyle, including her diet and exercise program. She lost forty pounds, so she did not need any liposuction after all. No one can sustain true

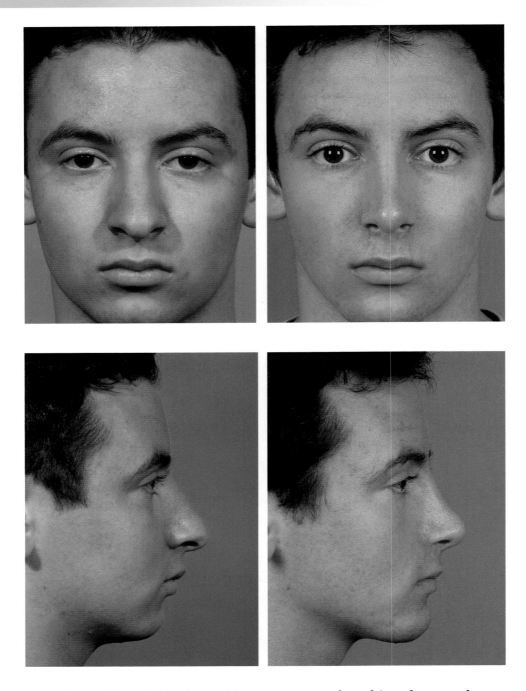

Dramatic facial and nasal improvement after rhinoplasty and chin augmentation

weight loss by surgery or liposuction alone; it takes a change of heart and mind, as well.

This is how I treat all of my patients, regardless of age. I look for the underlying core issues and evaluate the patient as a whole to see what is really going on in their lives before recommending a particular treatment. Surgery is sometimes part of this healing process, but often it is not, especially when the patient is still young. **Plastic surgery is not a miracle fix, nor should it be a crutch. As a committed professional, I see far further than the need for a sculpted nose or reshaped ears.**

The Invincible Twenties

Your twenties usher in a whole new set of aesthetic concerns. Young adults entering the work force for the first time want and need to look their best. Ideally, they become more conscious regarding their skin and wearing sunscreen. The more you protect and take care of skin now, the healthier you'll be later in life. The twenties are an era when life habits become fully established. These can include beneficial as well as harmful practices. The challenge for me as a doctor is to convince young adults to see beyond immediate gratification and take responsibility for their lives and bodies.

There are basic steps of preventative care that I emphasize: don't smoke, exercise frequently, adopt proper nutrition and great skin care, and of course, use sunscreen. Young people often feel invincible and live for the moment. I am here to tell you that you're *not* invincible and bad decisions can catch up to you eventually.

While prevention is always the best treatment, when damage has already been done, there are treatments and surgical options that can help. This is the time to begin the lifelong basic steps for true medical-grade skin care, which we'll discuss in detail in Chapter 4.

Operative procedures in this age group tend to be mostly for correcting congenital problems. Common procedures are breast augmentation and reduction, nose reshaping, and liposuction of diet-and-exercise-resistant areas (flanks, saddlebags, etc.). **But by far, the most popular procedures for people in their twenties are the non-invasive treatments, such as true medical skin care, which includes Retin-**

A® (Tretinoin), selective use of Botox® (onabotulinumtoxinA—a neuromodulator) and injectable fillers, laser skin resurfacing for acne scarring, microdermabrasion for improving skin tone, chemical peels and laser peels (for acne scars), laser hair removal, and laser treatment of leg veins. (We use Botox® and Retin-A® as general terms as they are more consumer recognizable, but these are brand names only for which there are numerous other similar medications available.)

We'll discuss each of these procedures in detail in later chapters. The main point at this young age, when most people are healthy and youthful looking, is prevention and correction. You want to start young with a great skin care regimen and follow it throughout life (see Chapter 4). If you haven't done this yet, no matter what your age is, it's never too late. **Plastic surgery is never a substitute for proper diet and exercise. You can't be doing tummy tucks by day and pizza by night! Your primary healthcare provider isn't your plastic surgeon. It's you!**

Mary is exactly right. Only you can take care of your own body. Sometimes that means taking steps to ensure proper diet and exercise. At other times, it means recognizing when surgery is necessary. This is an excellent time to begin taking responsibility for your appearance.

For example, about a year ago, one of my facelift patients brought her daughter Sheila to see me. Sheila was twenty-one and about to graduate from NYU. Since age ten, she had been unhappy with the bump on her nose, and she finally wanted to do something about it before entering the workforce. It was the perfect time for rhinoplasty because she had a month off before starting her new job in Washington, D.C. She is now one year post-op and her confidence level is completely transformed—she is still the same, only better. That is exactly what she told me when I removed her nasal splint at a week post-op as she looked into the mirror.

The Incredible Thirties

People in their thirties usually have begun to establish careers, marriages, and families, and they want to maintain their youthful appearance.

They may have started to notice creases around the brow and mouth, sun damage, spots, additional weight gain, and loss of facial fat as fat moves in a downward direction. New mothers may notice abdominal skin stretching and drooping after having children.

There are solutions. People in their thirties should still, first and foremost, focus on personal fitness, but there are other interventions and therapies that can augment their already healthy lifestyles. This is a time when patients may want to begin exploring injection therapies for the treatment of forehead, frown, and laugh lines. There are also post-

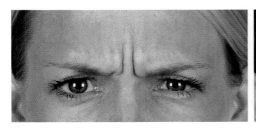
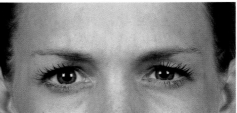
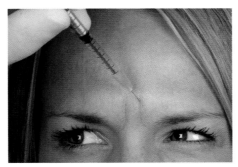

Classic treatment of frown lines with Botox® (onabotulinumtoxinA) injections in a 30-year-old female

pregnancy surgical procedures that can be done to lift or enhance the breasts, tighten the tummy, and reshape the hips and thighs. **Popular surgical procedures may include postpartum breast augmentation/lift or reduction, liposuction, microdermabrasion, chemical peel, laser treatment of leg veins, and tummy tucks (especially after having children).**

Still, the most popular procedures for people in their thirties continue to be the non-invasive ones, such as medical skin care and light-based treatments like IPL (also known as photofacial). These become more and more important with increased age and sun damage.

It is crucial that you have honest conversations with your surgeon to make sure that any procedures you undergo are carefully considered and age-appropriate. Too much of a neuromodulator like Botox®, for example, is generally not suitable for most people in their early thirties—most patients will need only minimal injections. It's also important to continue to practice excellent skin care, using medical-grade products—especially anti-aging agents like Retin-A®. (See Chapter 4)

I advise patients to have all of their children before they have a breast lift, tummy tuck, "mommy makeover," and/or any other body contouring or liposuction to avoid having your surgeon's careful work simply undone by the demands of pregnancy and childbirth. After you have had all of your children, though, you can be an ideal candidate for many of these procedures.

Kimberly, a thirty-five year-old patient, came to see me two years after her last child was born. Despite exercising five days a week, she was unable to get rid of her excess tummy skin from pregnancy. Breastfeeding her two children had also caused considerable loss of breast tissue. She was ready to get into better shape now that she was done having kids, but despite taking care of herself, she was struggling to get her old figure back. The reason was not lack of exercise or motivation—she was doing both. The problem was she had extra skin from pregnancy, and no amount of exercise or dieting was ever going to fix this!

She is now over two years post-op from a tummy tuck and tightening of her abdominal muscles as well as a breast augmentation. She remains in great shape. Diet and exercise were vital, but only the addition of body and breast contouring was enough to help restore Kimberly's previous body shape.

I had another patient in her thirties, Nancy, who went about the process all wrong. She always wanted to have fuller and fuller lips—so she went to a different practitioner and had her lips done. When I first saw her in consultation, her upper lip was larger than her lower lip. This is very unnatural and can give you an overdone Hollywood look or, worse, a primate-like appearance. (Giraffes and monkeys have larger upper than lower lips, but this does not look good in humans. Unfortunately, this is also true of some Hollywood stars whose names we won't mention.)

Nancy's work had clearly been done by someone with no real understanding of normal human anatomy, much less the finesse of a natural, youthful look. Fortunately, the practitioner had used a hyaluronic acid filler, which I reversed with hyaluronidase treatment (a medication used to melt away the filler over one to two days). Nancy now looks great and balanced. I see her yearly to keep her lips mildly and proportionately augmented until she is ready for any other age-appropriate procedures to continue to keep her looking great as she moves into her forties.

Nancy was lucky—this isn't always the case.

Jerri came to see me for the first time because her eyebrow had dropped after going overboard with Botox® and fillers. She had the work performed in her family doctor's office by an untrained medical assistant. In addition to the poorly done Botox®, she also had some unknown permanent fillers put into her face that were, she was told, "superb and long-lasting." The filler turned out to be adulterated, non-sterile industrial silicone, which required operative removal. Even with surgery, this permanent filler could not be totally removed, and it left her with a deformed lip—forever! I have been working with her for over two years to return her lips and face to normal, and while we have made progress, some of the damage is still visible.

This is an example of an uninformed and susceptible patient being preyed upon by an untrained or poorly trained individual. Sadly, this is not an uncommon occurrence. Our goal is to prevent you from being tempted to even think about making such an unwise decision as getting plastic surgery or other cosmetic procedures done at a salon, spa, or in a doctor's office unless the doctor is properly certified (more on these certifications in the next chapter). People who are **not** trained or qualified to perform these procedures can do you permanent harm.

The bottom line is this: **Your thirties are an age between eras. People in their thirties tend to be more aware of their skin and body changes than when they were in their twenties.** *They may want to begin using Botox® or fillers to soften the onset of wrinkles. Also, they may begin thinking about possible surgical procedures, especially if they've already had their children. This is a crucial time to do the research to obtain the best surgeon for your particular needs or wants. Strive for moderation while getting the best and most natural-looking results.*

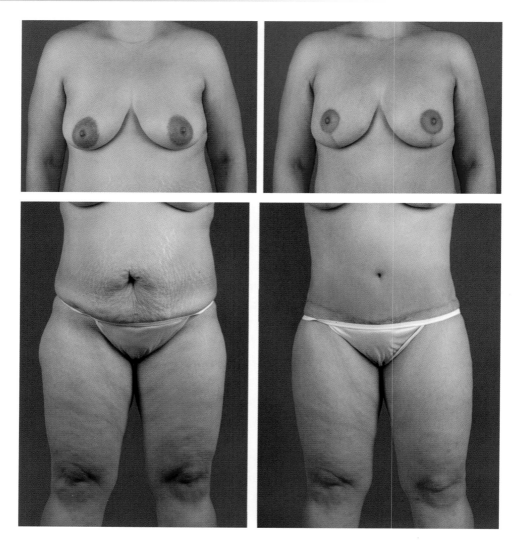

A "Mommy Makeover" patient with breast augmentation and lift with a tummy tuck and flank liposuction only

The Forties and Fifties (Let the Good Times Roll)

During your forties and through your mid-fifties, the aging process really begins to ramp up, and it may become increasingly difficult to maintain your appearance and health. **You may need to adjust your lifestyle to include more care and maintenance, adequate diet and exercise, and non-surgical technology and techniques. For many patients,** *this is also a time during which you will want to begin transitioning from fillers and Botox® to possible surgery, though this process will be gradual as you experience more and more facial aging.*

The eyes are called the "windows to the soul" because they are the most expressive of all facial features. That is why it is so **vital** not to change the appearance of your eyes too dramatically. Avoid excessive slanting or making them smaller with surgery, as this will forever change how you look and, for most patients, such changes are upsetting and undesirable. My patients want to look like themselves, only better. I am careful not to change the overall appearance or shape of their eyes.

In addition to facial work, people in this age group are more likely to want liposuction, tummy tucks, and other surgeries of the body—even with good diet and regular exercise, it can be hard to keep weight off of fat-prone areas, such as the hips in women and around the waist in men.

The main thing to understand about this phase of life is that it is another time of transition. (Are you seeing a pattern here? Change is ongoing!) We want you to understand and recognize when fillers and Botox® are just not enough to continue to make you look great, youthful, and natural. **You will eventually hit a point when these techniques alone may actually begin to make you look unnatural and older if they are overused! This is why you need an experienced plastic surgeon who knows how to do both fillers and surgery. You want your surgeon to be able to recognize when the fillers and Botox® are no longer cutting it and when it is time to transition to operative procedures so you can continue looking and feeling your best.**

The Glorious Sixties and Beyond—The Carefree Times (We Hope!)

In the past, people in this age group were often facing a slowdown in life as they approached retirement. Today, a later retirement is more and more common and professionals still want—and need—to look and feel their best. Even if you are an individual who wants and has the means to

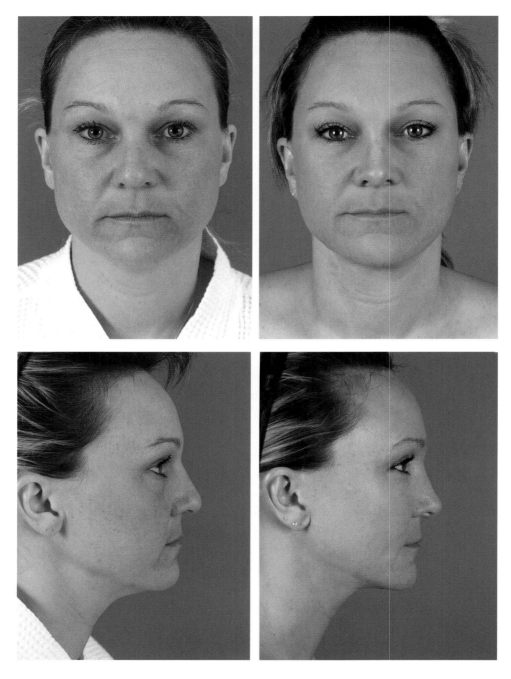

Early 40s' patient with facial rejuvenation (upper and lower eyelids and "Lift and Fill" facelift) to make her look as good as she feels

slow down and focus on personal passions, hobbies, and family, you still want to look and be the best you can. The desire to look and feel good about yourself transcends all age groups.

Patients in their sixties and beyond will have many of the same concerns as those in their forties and fifties, but those concerns are likely to be more pronounced. You may be more likely to want both face and body work at this age. **You might also explore surgical facial rejuvenation to bring back the natural jawline and reestablish the youthful fullness our cheeks had when we were younger. Again, it is best to seek a full facial rejuvenation approach for facial harmony, such as a face or neck lift, with your own fat used as a filler.** Fat makes the best filler in the mid-face or cheek areas for a natural look. More on the science behind this later.

In addition to these surgical procedures, the non-invasive techniques remain important. Medical-grade skin care, light-based treatments, injectables (fillers and Botox®), microdermabrasion, laser hair removal, IPL, chemical and skin resurfacing are all quite useful in this age group to complement surgery. These non-invasive treatments are, at this point, not primary treatments, but great supplements to reinforcing facial rejuvenation and body-contouring results.

The best time to begin considering surgery is when you start seeing the early signs of eye, face, and body aging (see computerized aging progression on page 39). If you notice hollowed eyes, sagging facial or neck skin, or fat accumulation in the neck, abdomen, or trunk areas—your time may be now! The earlier you treat, the better results you will see and the longer they will last. Also, there is absolutely no reason to put off addressing a current problem. You want to prevent others from even noticing that you are aging! The process is ongoing and so are the rewards. Why wait for improvements you could have now?

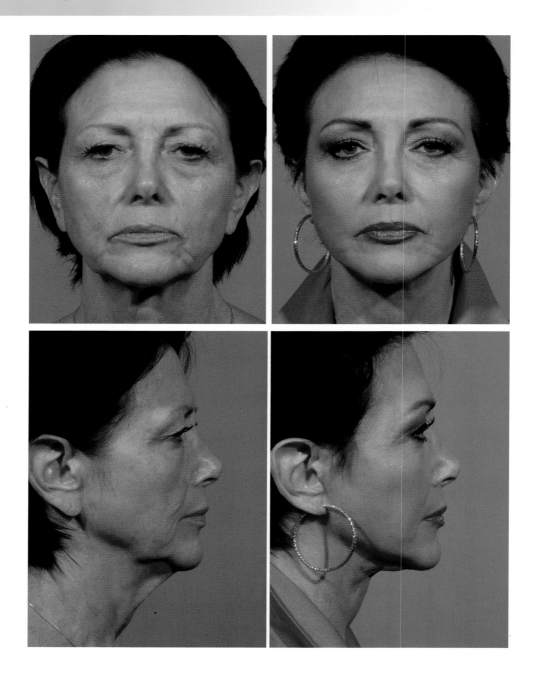

60s' facial rejuvenation ("Lift and Fill" facelift with eyelids) created more youthful fullness to cheeks and jawline as well as her eyes and lip areas

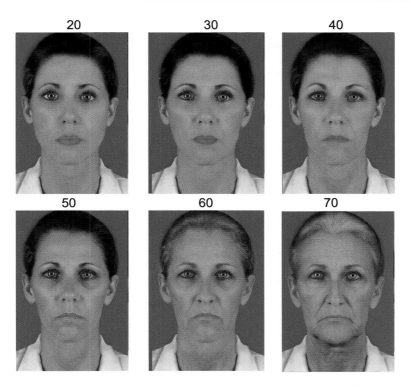

Computer simulation of age progression from the 20's to the 70's (front view)

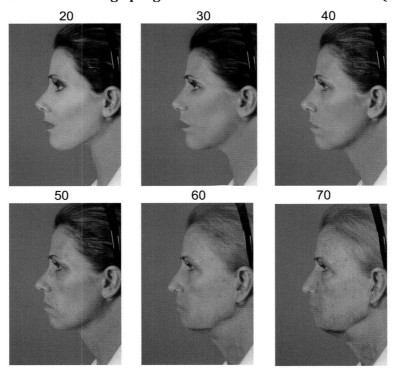

Computer simulation of age progression from the 20's to the 70's (side view)

Five Key Points to Remember:

1. Learn what is best for you at each stage in life. Practice great skin care no matter what your age.

2. Teens are vulnerable to criticism. Plastic surgery can help boost their self-confidence, especially if they have prominent ears, nasal deformities, and excessively enlarged breasts (in males or females).

3. Non-invasive procedures such as fillers and Botox® often work well to keep you looking great into your forties and early fifties.

4. Add operative procedures gradually, so you can maintain a natural and youthful look throughout your life.

5. Create a long-term plastic surgery plan with your plastic surgeon so you can continue to look as good as you feel for a long time—Navigate Your Beauty!

Finding and Consulting With Your Expert Plastic Surgeon

3

*We absolutely can't say this enough. If you take one thing from this book, let it be this: The first and most important decision you will make as a patient considering plastic surgery is your choice of surgeon. This is a very personal and also subjective matter that needs full attention and care. No one surgeon is perfect for every patient or procedure, and ultimately it is up to you to decide if a particular surgeon is right for you. You should trust your intuition and err on the side of caution. You don't just want a plastic surgeon; you want a **great** plastic surgeon.*

*The significant questions are: What makes a surgeon great? What makes a surgeon a true expert? We offer what we call the **Three Magic Questions** to ask so you can determine whether your surgeon is to be entrusted with your appearance ... and your health and well-being.*

To begin with, you will want to find someone who is both a verifiable expert in the particular procedure or procedures you are interested in and who possesses well-rounded experience throughout the field of plastic surgery. Your surgeon should have undergone extensive training and practice—__Expertise__ plus __Experience__ and __Exceptional results__ are what make an __Expert__ over the long term.

Actions always speak louder than words—or websites. Check for professional accomplishments beyond actual surgery. Focus on these three points, the *Three Magic Questions*, and limit your options for surgeons to those whose answers are positive. These questions will quickly help you determine whether you have a surgeon you should consider for your procedure. If the answer to any of these questions is no, buyer beware!!! Of course, all plastic surgeons need to be certified by the American Board of Plastic Surgery (ABPS), but that is just the beginning of finding the right plastic surgeon for you.

We offered you the **Three Magic Questions** as we began the book. Use these as a guide and they will not fail you. Here they are again, for your review:

1. **Is this one of the top three surgeries you perform and how often do you do it?** Choose a surgeon for whom this procedure is one of their top three, with a minimum of at least one of these procedures per week over the past five years. Now you know he or she has the **Experience** you demand for the procedure you want.

2. **Do you teach, speak, or write about this procedure for the benefit of other plastic surgeons?** The answer will quickly reveal the surgeon's level of **Expertise** in the procedure you desire.

3. **Do you have long-term follow-up photos for this procedure?** As the prospective patient, you should like the results you see. Insist on seeing/reviewing at least two or more long-term (greater than one year) patient results for the procedure you are considering. You need to see consistent, **Exceptional results** you really like.

In summary, you need to find the right plastic surgeon for you with the **Three C's (Caring, Compassionate, and Completely Empathetic), Three A's (Amiable, Available, and Able), and the *Three Magic Questions*: 1. Experience 2. Expertise 3. Exceptional Results.**

Three C's	Three A's
1. Caring	1. Amiable
2. Compassionate	2. Available
3. Completely Empathetic	3. Able

Key components of the right plastic surgeon for you

The best surgeons aren't always the easiest to find. Normally, they don't do mass marketing—they don't need that kind of thing, because they are in high demand thanks to their professionalism and reputation. The ***Three Magic Questions*** will not steer you wrong!

Three Magic Questions = Expert

1. Experience

2. Expertise

3. Exceptional Results

*For this chapter, Dr. Rohrich and I have assembled a Ten Point Checklist that you should use to evaluate a surgeon, along with a list of the **Three Magic Questions** you need to ask prospective surgeons. This list is not meant to be comprehensive. If you have a question, ask it! Your surgeon needs to know what your concerns are, and you need to know if you've got someone who will be empathetic and attuned to your needs.*

Keep notes on each prospective surgeon as you go. If at any time a surgeon doesn't measure up, look elsewhere. Do not feel pressured or forced to work with any particular surgeon, no matter how much time you spend with them in consultation. If you still have reservations at the end of the research process, trust your intuition and keep looking. Trust me, the right surgeon is out there for you.

Now, on to the list.

The Ten Point Checklist

1. **Your prospective surgeon should be board certified by the appropriate Specialty Group for the procedure you are contemplating.**

Specifically, your surgeon should be board certified by the American Board of Plastic Surgery (ABPS) or, if practicing in Canada, The Royal College of Physicians and Surgeons of Canada. Many patients fail to realize that a valid medical degree allows any doctor to legally perform medical procedures—a fact that should probably scare you! **Only doctors certified by the ABPS are recognized by the ABMS (American Board of Medical Specialties) as qualified to perform aesthetic surgical procedures.**

You can rest assured that a surgeon who is board certified by the ABPS will—at the very minimum—possess the following credentials:

- **Three to five years of training in general surgery and two to three years of training in plastic surgery.**

- **Successful completion of all written and oral tests administered by the ABPS (American Board of Plastic Surgery).**

- **Enrollment in ongoing continuing education, including rigorous written testing administered at least once every ten years, to ensure they stay current with new trends in the field.**

Visit the American Board of Medical Specialties website (http://www.abms.org/) to verify that your surgeon is properly board certified by the above agencies. Be wary of a surgeon who claims to be certified by another agency, no matter how professional the agency appears to be. There are a number of agencies of varying quality offering doctors "board certification" in plastic surgery. Some of these organizations have chosen names, often intentionally and with the intent to misrepresent, that sound very similar to the American Board of Plastic Surgeons (ABPS).

In general, accept no substitutes—this is the easiest way to be sure you are getting a fully licensed professional. However, there are exceptions you can make if you are willing to do the legwork to be sure they are qualified. **Patients receiving FDA-approved fillers or Botox® treat-**

ments can also choose a licensed medical doctor who is trained in one of the American Board of Medical Specialties (ABMS) core specialties (ophthalmology, dermatology, otolaryngology, plastic surgery). But again, such an M.D. must be trained in the use of fillers and Botox®. Be sure to ask about this. In addition, verify the information you receive by checking out the doctor's background and the work he or she has done on other patients. Ask to see photos and even speak to patients. If they don't look natural or normal—stop there and go elsewhere! (Ask the ***Three Magic Questions.***)

A patient considering cosmetic surgery of the face can also consider an M.D. who is a board certified otolaryngologist (ear, nose, and throat doctor) who specializes in facial plastic surgery—but only if they have the proven skills to do these procedures. They may operate on the head and neck areas only; never below the clavicle or neck area. **In general though, it is safest to go with an ABMS-certified surgeon (otolaryngologist or plastic surgeon) just to be on the safe side for facial cosmetic surgery.** The ABPS stamp of approval is your shorthand for a fully certified plastic surgeon for both face and body. Please remember this as it will get you into the correct group that is trained to do real plastic surgery.

An added perk of selecting a surgeon with proper certification is that you will be able to check his or her legal records and state medical board records. Most states will maintain records of any disciplinary actions and malpractice judgments filed against your perspective surgeon. These records can usually be found online. Even great plastic surgeons may have an attempted malpractice case filed against them, possibly filed frivolously and without due cause.

For example, during the so-called Great Breast Implant Crisis of the 1990s, a significant number of board certified plastic surgeons who performed breast augmentation were sued simply for performing silicone-implant breast augmentation. Not one plastic surgeon operating in the United States has ever, to my knowledge, been the target of a successful lawsuit just for putting in breast implants! These lawsuits were the result of the lack of conclusive medical data on the longevity of breast implants (all implants have an approximate lifespan of ten to fifteen years) and media reports that implants could cause cancer or autoimmune disease. These alleged reports have been scientifically disproved and breast implants today (both silicone and saline) are FDA-approved and safe.

Even responsible, skilled surgeons will sometimes be the targets of lawsuits, especially in the United States, in the absence of serious and comprehensive tort reform. Of course, you should take all such allegations seriously, making note of them—along with all other matters of concern—so that you remember to bring them up during consultation. Don't be afraid to be direct. **A good plastic surgeon will be open and honest about such incidences—if they aren't, you can and should continue your search elsewhere.**

2. Find references you can trust.

For references, it is best is to ask your personal physician, your friends in health care or those who work in great hospitals. They may know who is the best of the best in plastic surgery. Also, seek out your friends who have had plastic surgery and ask them ... especially if they look great themselves. The optimum result in plastic surgery is a situation where you don't even know if they had work done—they just look great and natural!

If numerous people refer you to the same doctor, he should make your top three list of board certified plastic surgeons to interview. **Next, check the Internet, as it is a powerful tool for researching plastic surgeons. Avoid relying solely on what you find online as this material is not vetted and may be misleading or inaccurate. As I mentioned earlier, everyone is famous on their own website.** Beware of advertisements and materials masquerading as unbiased reviews.

Visit the online forums where you can read legitimate patient reviews and accounts of patient experiences. **Keep in mind, however, that these websites can be deceptive and that *the Internet is replete with falsified good and bad patient reviews*.** Even legitimate online doctor rating systems can be manipulated. Some doctors hire search engine optimization (SEO) firms that actually fabricate patient reviews. These SEO firms are very good at getting around legitimate websites' fraud-prevention mechanisms—so you must beware of fake reviews even from trusted sites.

Also, be aware that not all bad reviews are warranted. It can actually be a red flag if a physician or surgeon has *only* great reviews—many search engines will discredit them, and so should you.

You need to seek advice from third parties that you can trust. When you first set out looking for a new surgeon, seek out references from family and friends who have undergone plastic surgery themselves as well as from trusted physicians. A good place to start is with your own primary care physician—even if they don't personally know any plastic surgeons, they may be able to refer you to a relevant specialist who can help.

3. Examine your prospective surgeon's website.

When doing a web search of your prospective surgeon's name, you will find that their personal website will probably be one of the top hits. Be sure to look it over carefully. This is the most direct way to find well-organized information about your prospective surgeon all in one place. It is a place for valuable information—so use it.
Start with the bio page to get a sense of their experience and approach to medical practice. Do they mention patient care? Aftercare? Great care begins before a surgery and ends only after recovery. A surgeon who focuses only on performing surgery may be more interested in selling you surgery than providing you with total care. If the website seems less interested in being informative about the procedures offered than it is about selling you a procedure, run the other way.

While a physician's website can be a great place to conduct preliminary research, websites can also be carefully curated and designed to convince you of a surgeon's considerable competence, whether or not such distinction is deserved. One of the most common things I hear from rhinoplasty and facelift patients who have suffered deformities at the hands of unqualified surgeons is this: "But the doctor had a great website and a lot of certificates hung on their office walls." Unfortunately, these patients failed to read what these certificates actually stated, to understand who granted them and with what authority, and whether the surgeon was vetted by a legitimate authority, preferably the ABMS.

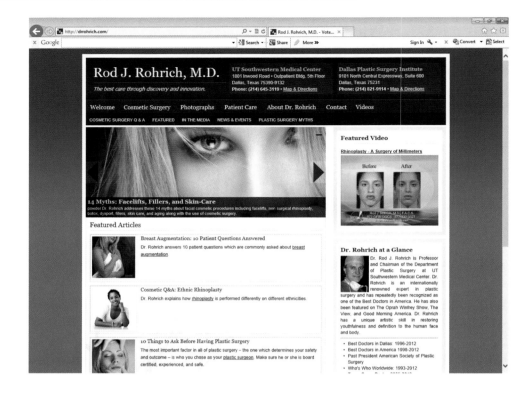

Home page of Dr. Rohrich's website

*As a patient considering plastic surgery, I found the Internet to be a re-markably useful tool for doing research for a prospective surgeon. **How-ever, I was also cautious and guarded, as I know the Internet does not have quality filters! Use the Internet to screen out those doctors who don't meet the criteria we have suggested. I often found most useful and interesting the before-and-after pictures of patients.** Keep in mind, though, that these photos often represent the surgeon's best work, captured in the most flattering angle and lighting, and there is always the possibility that the photos may have been doctored (no pun intended!). Ask to see recent photographs during your consultation, be-cause websites are not always updated as regularly as they should be and the photographs online may be out of date.*

4. Verify that your prospective surgeon has hospital privileges.

"Hospital privileges" refers to the right of a physician to use the equipment and facilities of a given hospital. Even if you are undergoing an outpatient procedure, your surgeon still needs to have hospital privileges. Hospitals that are accredited within the United States employ credential committees to perform extensive background checks on surgeons before extending hospital privileges. **Hospital privileges indicate that surgeons have been vetted by their peers and by a hospital committee. It should be a red flag if your prospective plastic surgeon does not have hospital operating privileges.**

Furthermore, if you have a problem after surgery, you may need to be seen or admitted to a hospital. It is important that your surgeon can see you and treat you there.

5. Inquire about your surgeon's specific <u>experience</u>.

Once you have done your homework, you will be ready to meet the most promising of prospective surgeons face-to-face. Don't be afraid to ask questions. You will be entrusting this person with your face and/or body. **You have every right to make sure that this surgeon is right for you, possessing the experience and expertise they claim. Do they do this procedure at least once a week and is it one of the top three procedures they do? (*Three Magic Questions*)**

While you are in consultation, try to get a sense of what their work experience includes and, just as importantly, how they work. Follow up on all of the things you looked into online, filling in any holes and forming a whole picture of them as a physician, a surgeon, and a person. In short, make a comprehensive list of questions. No question is too dumb or tedious, and if a medical provider treats your questions as such, walk away. You aren't auditioning for the role of patient!

6. Ask your prospective surgeon to clarify all potential benefits, risks, and complications.

All surgery is real surgery and should not be entered into haphazardly. Plastic surgery, like any other surgical procedure, may produce real complications, albeit relatively rare when performed by a competent surgeon. You should not let undue fear make your choices for you, but great surgeons take these risks seriously ... and so should you.

Plastic surgery is very safe in healthy patients who have no major medical problems and do not smoke. However, as with any surgery, there are potential risks of infection, bleeding, excess scarring, no improvement, a need for revision surgery, damage to blood vessels and nerves, and asymmetry. Very infrequently there is the risk of blood clots and even death in very rare instances.

Your plastic surgeon should be readily forthcoming with information about risks and potential complications. Some of these will be specific to your procedure and others will be furthermore specific to you. Be sure that your surgeon is aware of any relevant medical conditions, current prescriptions, drug allergies, and relevant lifestyle choices, such as smoking or drinking alcohol, that might be contraindicated for certain surgeries and that could affect your outcome or care.

*Remember that plastic surgery almost always involves elective procedures. You are free to opt out at any time, for any reason. You may find in the course of your research that the procedure you were considering is not right for you. That's okay. That too can be a part of the process. It's your journey, and you get to navigate your beauty as you see fit. **You shouldn't have any procedure or surgery unless you are 100 percent sure in your decision. Once you have decided on the right plastic surgeon for you, everything becomes so much clearer and easier.***

Mary is correct. A surgeon should never make you feel pressured or rushed about such an important decision. Any pressure at all is, in fact, a sign that you should reconsider working with the offending surgeon. The desire to look younger, thinner, or more beautiful can leave you particularly susceptible to influence or manipulation. You don't want to be paranoid, but you should remain vigilant and on guard.

Be extremely wary of discounts offered for plastic surgery. By all means, shop around, but prices that are far below market value should be alarming. We call these **"bottom feeders."** They attract patients with lower fees. Fees significantly below market rates are a red flag!

Don't take chances with something as important as your own body just for the chance to save a little (or even a lot) of money, and you should never settle for subpar work. Remember, in medicine, as in life, you generally get what you pay for, and if it sounds too good to be true, it probably is.

7. **When it comes time for your surgery, it should be performed in an accredited ambulatory facility. (Staying Safe)**

These facilities are subject to review by both internal staff and outside inspectors. An ambulatory facility will have the equipment and personnel to respond quickly and effectively to any emergency that may arise during the course of your procedure. Plastic surgery, when performed by a great surgeon, is generally safe. Here's a great secret that you need to know: **If you choose a board certified plastic surgeon who is a member of ASPS (American Society of Plastic Surgery) or ASAPS (American Society for Aesthetic Plastic Surgery), which are the largest plastic surgery organizations with only board certified plastic surgeons—he or she is mandated to operate only in accredited ambulatory OR facilities.**

A surgeon who has access to an ambulatory facility has undergone outside peer review to do so—similar to a surgeon who has attained hospital privileges. The more vetted your surgeon is, the better. ***Most cosmetic surgery is not performed as an inpatient procedure, but it should at least be performed at an accredited ambulatory facility in order to better ensure your safety with good post-op nursing care facilities.***

8. **A great surgeon will employ a carefully selected and certified anesthetist or anesthesiologist.**

This is the person who will administer your anesthesia. An *anesthetist* is a nurse while an *anesthesiologist* is a medical doctor. Either can provide wonderful care, but only if they possess the necessary experience and expertise. Be sure that they are certified to administer anesthesia, whether they are an anesthesiologist or a certified registered nurse anesthetist (CRNA). This means they've been certified with strict criteria after completing several years of training beyond their M.D. or R.N. degree.

Many patients are anxious about receiving general anesthesia as it is one of the most misunderstood parts of having cosmetic surgery. Modern anesthesia is very safe unless it is administered poorly or because of a very rare idiosyncratic patient response to anesthetic. The key is to have a dedicated, qualified person administer your anesthesia, and this is not your plastic surgeon.

Having selected a certified ambulatory facility or accredited hospital operating room for your procedure ensures that, in the *unlikely* event of an emergency, your surgical team will have the backup and equipment and expertise necessary to help ensure your safety.

You should meet with your anesthesiologist before your surgery. I have my anesthesiologists call patients the night before surgery to review what they will be doing and go over any last-minute questions. Both the anesthesiologist and I meet again with the patient on the morning of the procedure to review all the risks and benefits once more.

9. Discuss your recovery period with your prospective surgeon.

Just as a great surgeon will work with you during the lead-up to your surgery, they will also understand that their patients remain their patients throughout the recovery process. Of special importance is the first 24 to 48 hours after surgery, and you will want to discuss this period in detail so you know what to expect, how to identify problems, how to care for yourself, and when to follow up with your physician or another medical professional.

This is crucial whether going home right after surgery or being transferred to a post-operative facility. You may even want to pay extra attention as an outpatient, as you will need to be able to identify problems and administer your own post-operative care. For example, a certain amount of discomfort can be expected while your body heals after many surgical procedures. You need to know what is a normal amount of discomfort when your body heals and what might represent pain from a complication, such as infection.

Every procedure comes with its own risks. You will want to know what possible complications may arise and how to deal with them if they do—the risk of specific complications will vary depending on the details of your procedure and specific circumstances.

Just as every patient's surgery is unique, so too is every recovery. You will want to know when you are realistically going to be able to return to work, exercise, and your regular daily routine. Discuss any particularities about your lifestyle with your surgeon—if you want to know when you will be able to get back to your triathlon training, for example, you need to ask! Otherwise, how will your surgeon be aware of your unique needs? Communication and established trust are always key.

For much more information on aftercare and recovery, please see Chapter 12.

10. **Get additional opinions from appropriate professionals, if needed or desired.**

Once you have finally settled on a particular surgeon, it may be prudent to consider seeking a second—or even third—opinion from other board certified plastic surgeons. This is especially true if you have concerns or have further questions that were not answered to your satisfaction. I always tell my new patients to come back or email, call, or text me after the consultation if there is something they forgot to ask or I didn't answer during the consultation.

Bring your notes with you to your consultation. If you have specific concerns about your prospective surgeon, voice them right then. As Mary pointed out earlier, don't be afraid to change your mind at any point, no matter how far along you are in the process.

The choice of surgeon is a very personal and subjective decision and one that only you get to make. This is your body, your procedure. Any reason to select a different surgeon is good enough; you may simply have a better rapport with one surgeon than another. Remember, expertise and experi-

ence are everything—and should never be discounted. Ensure that your goals and your surgeon's goals are in line with one another and also that they are realistic.

Mary makes another excellent point here—a great surgeon will let you know if your goals and desired outcome are possibly unrealistic or overly optimistic.

No amount of plastic surgery, for example, will make you look like you did when you were thirty years old if you are now seventy; a more realistic goal is to make you look the best you can for your age. A great surgeon will work with you to assist you in deciding what your goals are and how best to achieve them—sometimes this will involve the procedure you first wanted, and sometimes it will not. Keep an open mind.

So there you have it—our Ten Point Checklist for finding a great plastic surgeon. We cannot stress enough how important the above criteria are, and we urge you to approach this choice as an ongoing process with which you must remain engaged. One last cautionary tale, to keep you on your toes as you research your options:

A new patient came to see me about a botched facelift surgery, performed by a non-board certified surgeon in a non-accredited operating room that had resulted in unsightly loss of skin in front of and behind her ear and a facial nerve injury that resulted in a droopy exposed eyelid and paralysis of her entire cheek and lip area, so much so that saliva drooled out of her mouth for almost six months. Not a pretty sight for a previously beautiful woman. We had to wait a full year for her wounds to heal before I could even begin reconstructing her face. The non-board certified surgeon had been mass-marketing online at a bargain basement price. That should have been the first red flag!

The second red flag should have gone up when her surgeon failed to see her or prepare her at her pre-op consultation. Her operation was performed as an outpatient procedure in his office (non-accredited operating facility) with only local anesthetic used—a third and major red flag! A fourth and final flag probably would have gone up in a post-op consultation, but her surgeon didn't follow through here and see her post-op, either—in fact, he has since fled the country! The patient was an intelligent woman but did not know what questions to ask. We want to help prevent this from happening to you!

This patient could have saved herself a great deal of pain and suffering by being aware of the many warning signs—don't let her mistakes also be yours. The risks of picking the wrong surgeon are far too dire, and even a very basic amount of research can prevent some such tragedies. Be a proactive patient and actually do the research.

This is a pretty scary story. Dr. Rohrich's purpose in telling this story is to show you what can really happen if you fail to do your research before picking a plastic surgeon. He is trying to prevent you from falling prey and becoming a statistic. Use this book as your guide and you will be well and properly prepared. I did my research, asked the questions, and found a great plastic surgeon, and so can you!

The Consultation—Coming Prepared and Informed

Once you have settled on a prospective surgeon, you can begin thinking about the initial consultation. During your first meeting, you should learn as much as you can about the surgeon as well as the actual procedure you are considering. **This time is also for the surgeon to get to know *you*—your wishes, your history, your medical status, your body type, and your surgical goals. Good plastic surgeons will not just schedule you for surgery. They will assess your situation and honestly ascertain whether or not they will be able to help you achieve your desires.**

Do the Mirror Test: Look in the mirror and identify the top three surgical priorities and/or changes you want made. Write these down and bring them with you to the initial consultation so you can get firm, immediate feedback and answers to any questions. Be as specific as you can in your questions, but don't be too aggressive—that can make it difficult for you and your surgeon to work together. Even the best plastic surgeon has limits. Take the case of a recent prospective patient I met; she set up a slideshow of her life story (fifty photos!) in order to give me "background" for her rhinoplasty—that was a little much. It is of the utmost importance that both of you are on the same page about all aspects of your procedure and recovery.

It is normal to have fears and anxieties. Discuss them with your surgeon at the consultation. Making the decision to have plastic surgery is transformative and exciting, but such excitement induces a certain amount of apprehension and you need to discuss every detail. Make sure to talk about the emotional aspects of your chosen procedure: what to expect now, after surgery, and in the months of healing to come. Open communication with your surgeon is key.

Some patients fear that pain and anxiety medications can be habit-forming. Typical treatment with plastic surgery is not long enough to lead to addiction. Special care is taken with those who have had substance abuse issues, and this is a plan of action that can be personalized with you and your doctor.

Mary and I have compiled a quick checklist to help prepare you for the first consultation. You will want to add your own questions to this list—particularly questions that are specific to your desired procedure (see the relevant chapters for more information)—but here are basic questions to get you started, all of which you will want answered:

THE CONSULTATION

TEN POINT CHECKLIST

1. Are you board certified by the American Board of Plastic Surgery (ABPS) or the American Board of Medical Specialties (ABMS) for the procedure(s) I desire?

2. Do you operate in an accredited operating facility? (If they are members of ASPS or ASAPS, they are required to do so.)

3. Are you an expert in this particular procedure? (Ask the **Three Magic Questions** to verify their answer—Experience, Expertise, and Excellent results.)

4. What are the most common risks and complications you have had with this procedure?

5. Can you tell me what to expect pre-op and post-op?

6. When will I look normal again? When can I return to work, my normal daily routine and exercise?

7. Can I see images of what I may potentially look like after my surgery?

8. Who is administering my anesthesia? (They must be a certified registered nurse anesthetist [CRNA] or board certified anesthesiologist.)

9. What if I have a problem or complication? Whom do I call and where do you see me?

10. If I need revision surgery, what will the cost be? Will you charge me? (You will most likely be responsible for the anesthesia and operating room costs. You need to know all of this upfront.)

The *THREE MAGIC QUESTIONS*

1. **Is this one of the top three surgeries you perform and how often do you do it?** Choose a surgeon for whom this procedure is one of their top three, with a minimum of at least one of these procedures per week over the past five years. Now you know he or she has the **Experience** you demand for the procedure you want.

2. **Do you teach, speak, or write about this procedure for the benefit of other plastic surgeons?** The answer will quickly reveal the surgeon's level of **Expertise** and respect by his peers in the procedure you desire.

3. **Do you have long-term follow-up photos for this procedure?** As the prospective patient, you should like the results you see. Insist on seeing/reviewing at least two or more long-term (more than one year) patient results for the procedure you are considering. You need to see consistent, **Exceptional results** you really like.

As a patient, you are also a consumer, so it is your right—and your responsibility—to prepare for the consultation. I wouldn't say that the surgeon so much works "on" you as works "with" you, so treat this as a true relationship. You will be seeing a lot of this person, so choose someone you really enjoy speaking to. Know as much as you can before consultation so you can learn as much in consultation. You will have a limited amount of time when meeting in the office, so you want to have the basics already covered.

So, while the consultation is a learning experience, do yourself a favor and come in having done foundational homework. Being informed allows for a more comprehensive and meaningful first meeting and will help you ensure that you have found a great surgeon that is a true expert in the procedure or procedures you desire. Take all the notes you can. It may feel stressful, but you'd be amazed at how much information people don't re-member from their consultations! The more information you write down, the better a decision you'll be able to make down the road.

Five Key Points to Remember:

1. Choosing a surgeon is the first and most important decision you will make when navigating your beauty. Research surgeons thoroughly and choose carefully.

2. Use the Ten Point Checklist to find a true expert who is a competent and qualified surgeon. You can use our checklist to take with you to the consultation.

3. Find a true plastic surgery expert for your specific procedure(s) by asking the **Three Magic Questions** to ensure the Experience, Expertise, and Exceptional results for the exact procedure(s) you want.

4. Know before you go—this means *doing your research first*. Be prepared and know what to expect and more importantly what to ask. (Your top three concerns.)

5. Remember that everyone is famous on their own website! Verify claims through independent research and second opinions.

Looking Great Without Plastic Surgery

How Skin Care and Skin Resurfacing
Make the Difference

4

Beauty may only be skin deep, as the expression goes, but maximizing the natural beauty of your skin requires digging deeply into the science of total skin care. That's the focus of this chapter. We are going to cover both what you can do at home and what your selected plastic surgeon can do to help.

Let's start by discussing the Five Keys to Good Skin Care.

The number of skin care products on the market can be bewildering. To simplify things, you want products with ingredients that have been proven effective. Here's what we recommend:

1. **Cleansers and Hydrators**—cleanse and hydrate daily with a gentle cleanser (pH neutral) and hydrator. You want to keep your skin supple, but also remove impurities.

2. **Exfoliators**—these products assist in the removal of dead skin cells from the outer layer of your skin, improving its look and feel. I prefer formulas composed of up to 10 percent alpha and/or beta hydroxy fruit acids, which help turn over the cells on the skin's outer layer only.

3. **Pigment Controllers**—such as hydroquinone and kojic acid, brighten the skin and reverse mild to moderate hyperpigmentation and sun damage. Pigment controllers such as these will even out your overall skin tone. Selective use is recommended depending upon your skin pigmentation problems.

4. **Anti-aging/Restorative Agents—Retin-A® (Tretinoin) and retinols are a topical retinoid derived from Vitamin A** that is scientifically proven to improve aging skin. It works by accelerating the process by which your skin cells turn over. Skin cells normally turn over every six weeks on average, but with the use of Retin-A®, this process only takes approximately six days. This faster turnover will improve the look and feel of skin by reducing the appearance of wrinkles and fine lines as well as evening out skin tone.

Some patients complain that Retin-A® and retinols induce reactions, such as irritation, flaking, and redness. In most cases, these side effects are not the result of an allergy, but are simply a normal part of acclimating to rapid skin cell turnover. If you experience these side effects, they normally subside within four to six weeks as your skin adjusts to the rejuvenation process. Those with oily skin may find that they can begin using Retin-A® every night. The rest will have to work their way up, increasing frequency of application and potency of the formula over time.

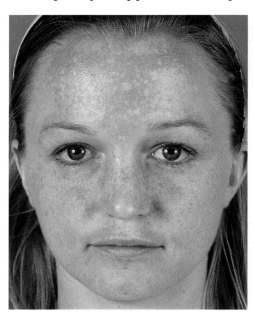 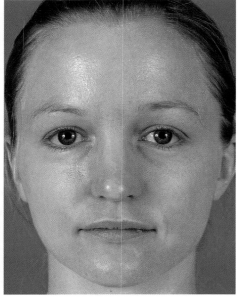

**Overall skin tone dramatically improved with long term use of
Retin-A® only (Trentinoin)**

5 Keys to Good Skincare

1. CLEANSERS AND HYDRATORS - PH neutral, remove impurities, oil and makeup, and use a daily hydrator to make skin more supple and enhance overall tone.

2. EXFOLIATORS - Remove dead skin cells by chemical or mechanical process and improve skin tone. Examples include fruit acid peels, skin scrubs, and skin brushes especially if you have thick, oily skin.

3. PIGMENT CONTROLLERS - Occasional use of pigment controllers even out overall skin tone and pigment. Examples are kojic acid and hydroquinone.

4. ANTI-AGING/RESTORATIVE AGENTS - Retin-A® (Tretinoin) turns over your outer skin cells faster, rejuvenating your skin within a matter of months, and can actually eliminate or reduce the appearance of wrinkles over time. Topical Vitamin C is an anti-oxidant that is useful to help repair and restore sun damaged skin.

5. PROTECTIVE AGENTS - Sunscreens will protect your skin from the damaging rays from the sun. Your sunscreen should be at least an SPF of 30 or higher and protect against UVA and UVB rays.

Another anti-aging agent is **Topical Vitamin C**, which is an antioxidant and useful to repair and restore sun damaged skin. The effect of free radicals can be offset through the use of oral antioxidants, such as Vitamin C.

5. **Protective Agents**—sunscreens will do more to protect your skin and keep it looking as youthful as you age. Your sunscreen should be SPF 30 or higher and protect against both UVA and UVB rays. UVA rays can prematurely age the skin while UVB rays can burn the skin—both result in lasting skin damage.

Your sunscreen should have either a chemical or physical barrier component. Sunscreens providing physical barriers (such as zinc or titanium) block the sun's damaging rays and also cause fewer rashes and allergies than chemical blockers.

Your face is the first thing people notice about you, and you want to keep it looking its best. **Beautiful skin starts with knowing the Five Keys to Good Skin Care and applying them consistently over the course of your lifetime. Basic skin care is something you should commit to long before there is ever a need for Botox®, fillers, or even surgery. Refer to this chart, which simplifies the five basic steps we discussed above.**

Understanding Your Skin

The skin is the body's largest organ, comprising 16 percent of your total body weight and measuring two square meters of surface area. The tone and texture of skin varies greatly depending on area of the body, thickness, and exposure to the elements. The outer layer of the skin is

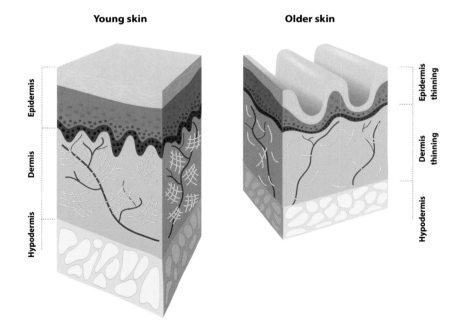

Thinning of skin layers with aging

responsible for our skin color (pigmentation) and protects us from the sun's damaging ultraviolet rays.

Our skin becomes thinner and less supple as we age. There are observable changes in all layers of skin—not only the outermost layer or epidermis. The reticular dermis is a deeper, thicker layer. Most people only pay attention to the outermost layer, not the deeper layers beneath the surface. They don't understand that this deeper, thicker layer also thins over time, contributing to aging by affecting the overlying visible layers. Ideally, we would like to halt the aging process before it affects the epidermis.

Thoughts About Rapid Skin Care

Rapid skin care is exactly what it sounds like—a medical-grade skin care technique that provides rapid results. Unlike the above skin care products that can be used at home, these rapid techniques require a professional. Your physician will literally remove the old outer layer of skin through one of three techniques:

1. *Dermabrasion*—involves sanding the skin.

2. *Chemical peel*—uses chemicals to remove the outer layer.

3. *Erbium laser peel*—uses a direct laser beam which removes the outer layer of skin without burning.

All of these methods work by the same basic mechanism: They injure and remove the outer layer of skin so that new skin can regenerate. "Injuring" the skin, put simply, is the process of removing old skin to make way for the new. The injury or effect needs to be confined to the dermis to have a visible effect on the skin. If the injury extends into the reticular (deeper) dermis, there is an increased risk of scarring. However, because deep wrinkles extend deeper into the skin, deeper treatments are sometimes necessary. You will only want an expert to perform deep treatments in order to minimize the risk of scarring.

Because different methods of injury penetrate the skin at different depths, some methods are better suited for specific situations. Of these three methods, I prefer a non-burning Erbium laser for wrinkle correction. **This laser provides a more consistent, uniform correction of deeper wrinkles than the other methods.** There are new lasers that penetrate your skin in specific, contained areas (commonly known as **fractional laser**), leaving the intervening skin unaffected. This allows you to treat twenty to thirty percent of the skin at a time and makes this technique ideal for spot treatment. This laser treats wrinkles directly by going deeper into the skin. Recovery time is approximately five to seven days. Erbium lasers, in my experience, are more precise than their predecessors and have less problems with hyperpigmentation if done properly by an experienced laser expert.

Chemical peels are the preferred treatment of choice for patients who have fine to moderate lines, but this method does require your plastic surgeon to have more control, expertise, and finesse. The peel basically etches off layers of the skin down to the

Chemical peels can:

- Repair uneven skin tone

- Revitalize and rejuvenate the skin

- Repair fine lines

- Reduce hyperpigmentation, acne marks, and sunspots

- Brighten the skin

- Treat sun damage

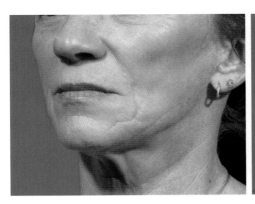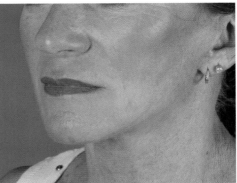

Patient with remarkable improvement from TCA peel around the mouth with a "Lift and Fill" facelift

middle layer of the dermis. (If you desire to go more deeply, you will need to employ one of the laser treatments.) A deeper peel requires twelve to fourteen days of downtime.

The key to a successful chemical peel is in the application. It's done with a trichloroacetic acid (TCA). In essence, a chemical peel is a superficial burn performed in a very gentle and controlled fashion. A chemical peel can be done on the entire face or on the area around the mouth. While you can also get into the neck area, peels in this area must stay very superficial.

A TCA peel can be light, moderate, or deep. A light peel can last anywhere from six to nine months, whereas moderate and deep peels can last for one to two years. TCA peels are deeper than glycolic or lactic acid peels. TCA peels are great for the face, the neck, and the back of your hands. If you have very sensitive skin, your surgeon should avoid the TCA peel as there are lighter peels that can be done by a skin care specialist.

Consult your surgeon on how to best prepare for your chemical peel. Your surgeon will probably have you discontinue any use of exfoliants, retinoids, or bleaching creams approximately one to two weeks before your peel. This will allow your skin sufficient time to rest before the deeper peel.

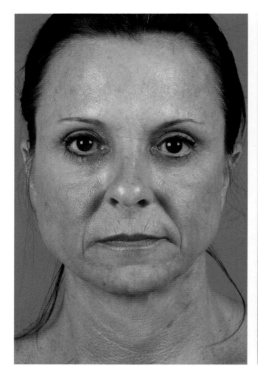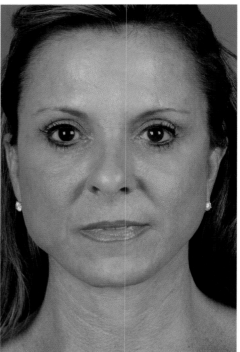

Dramatic improvement with a "Lift and Fill" facial rejuvenation, central facial TCA peel, and Erbium laser around the mouth

Gradual Skin Care

Some peels are available for at-home, do-it-yourself application, but they can be dangerous if not done properly. At-home peels only remove the uppermost superficial skin layers, and not the deeper layers, and do not have the same long-lasting results. They can, however, make your skin look and feel better and enhance overall skin tone temporarily.

There are three gradual skin care methods:

1. *Microdermabrasion* **is a mechanical process that sands the skin.** This is used only for removal of the outermost layer of the skin and, while useful, only provides superficial results.

Skin Care Solutions	
Skin Problem	Solution
Red Spots	IPL Treatments
Lines and Wrinkles	Retin-A®, Peels and Laser
Brown Spots	Retin-A®, IPL, Peels and Laser

2. *Alpha hydroxy peels* **are exceedingly common. They've been used since the times of ancient Egypt and are basically the tartaric acid of fermented wine.** The most common forms come from glycolic or lactic acid (no need to remember those terms), and they produce a light frost of rapid exfoliation and mild shedding for about two to three days. You might have heard of the "Lunchtime Peel"—this utilizes Jessner's solution and is a common example of a beta hydroxy peel.

3. *Intense pulsed light (IPL)*, **also known as photofacial, is available with a broad array of electromagnetic waves.** It's useful for some dyschromias (skin discolorations) and correcting redness. This usually requires a series of five treatments over three weeks, which will diminish sunspots and redness in the skin. Perhaps the greatest advantage of IPL is that it is safe for use in the neck, upper chest, and hands.

The Most Effective Ancillary Procedures

There are several other ancillary procedures patients use. These include the following:

- **Laser hair removal:** This is the removal of unwanted hair by exposure to pulses of laser light. This is most suitable for patients with coarse, dark, body hair and light skin, though new lasers now work for patients with other hair and skin tones, although less effectively. You will need several treatments, but this laser can provide long-lasting results.

- **Permanent Makeup:** This involves dying/tattooing the skin to apply permanent makeup. This can cosmetically enhance the lips, eyebrows, and eyes. These procedures need to be performed by **highly skilled** skin care professionals only.

- **Lymphatic Massage:** This specialized type of massage is good for post-surgery therapy as a way to decrease swelling, increase lymphatic circulation, and promote drainage of fluids from inflamed tissue.

- **Sclerotherapy:** Varicose and spider veins can be treated with FDA approved injectable agents or hypertonic saline(salt water). Please Verify that the injector has expertise in this area.

We realize the above is a lot of information to take in. Simply understand that you have many options at your disposal and discuss them with your surgeon. As you can see, there are a wonderful variety of treatments available and at least one will be well suited for you. For every procedure, it is vital that you recognize the importance of your own face, skin, genetics, and aging—complete navigated care.

Five Key Points to Remember:

1. Great skin care is essential and is a process to maintain throughout your life.

2. Medical-grade skin care means using the Five Keys to Good Skin Care.

3. Combine at-home gradual skin care with physician-assisted rapid skin care for best results.

4. IPL, microdermabrasion, fruit acid peels, and facials are great and safe ways to make your skin look good in the short term—use them regularly under the direction of your skin care expert.

5. For moderately deep wrinkles and fine lines, you may want to go with a chemical peel, such as a TCA peel. For deeper, permanent lines or wrinkles, you may want to use a specialized non-burning laser like the Erbium.

Knowing the Differences—Fillers, Botox®, and Your Own Fat

5

We have all seen the Hollywood types in the gossip magazines who have been done a real disservice by practitioners or doctors who sometimes call themselves plastic surgeons! Their great looks were marred, instead of enhanced, by procedures that went wrong. In my practice, I see patients like this all the time. Why did these stars, for whom appearance is everything, not put more time and effort into finding the right surgeon in whom to trust with their appearance? These highly visible cases of bad cosmetic surgery have unfairly given the field of plastic surgery a bad name. We don't notice the good cases of plastic surgery because the best plastic surgery is the kind you don't notice.

One of the most common causes of the dreaded "Hollywood Look" is the overuse and misuse of fillers to address sagging, for which they are not indicated. So in this chapter we will explore the different kinds of fillers, Botox® and one's own facial fat. Let's address what these can and cannot do for you.

Knowing the differences-Fillers, Botox® (onabotulinumtoxinA), and Your Own Fat

Fillers are used to add volume to your face when you have volume loss, but have not yet reached the point of sagging. Once sagging sets in, fillers won't do. **One of the most common mistakes that inexperienced physicians and other practitioners make is in the excessive promotion of these products, believing fillers can lift and fill for an easy fix.** They cannot. When overused, they create a very over-filled and fake appearance. *Fillers fill, but they do not lift effectively.* Anyone who suggests otherwise is doing you a disservice. Why do patients let this happen to them? Possibly because fillers do not require surgery and can be done more quickly and with less planning and commitment—just because a procedure doesn't require surgery doesn't mean it is easy or safe.

I recently received an urgent call from a distraught patient. She had a filler placed in her lower eyelid tear trough area, and it looked like a sausage under her eyelid. She was frantic because her son's wedding was in just five days. I saw her that day and discovered that a spa employee had injected her with an FDA-approved hyaluronic acid filler. This is a great filler for lips, but not for eyelids, as it can cause more tissue swelling in this area and absorbs water.

Luckily, since it was a hyaluronic acid filler, which is water-soluble, the effect was reversible. I used hyaluronidase, a medication that melts away the hyaluronic acid fillers (HA), and within 24 hours she looked the way she did before the injection. She made it to the wedding looking great, and she was very fortunate. **The lesson: Make sure you're getting the right filler in the right place and that you're in the hands of a board certified plastic surgeon, dermatologist, facial plastic surgeon (ENT), or oculoplastic surgeon who is well-versed in the use of the filler you're considering. Don't allow someone just working in a spa and not professionally trained to inject anything into you!**

Once again, fillers fill, but they do not lift. As the face begins to sag, because of lost volume, it may be time to consider surgery. If sagging is not a problem, then fillers can be wonderful tools to fill out and re-volumize your face without the invasiveness or the expense of surgery.

When it comes to FDA-approved fillers in the USA, you have many options. The seven most commonly used fillers are the following:

1. *Restylane® and Perlane®*—hyaluronic acid occurs naturally in our bodies and aids in regulating growth and cell renewal—these are excellent hyaluronic acid fillers that are great for filling the cheek, nasolabial folds, under the eyes (tear troughs), and the lower jaw (chin) areas. They usually last more than six months, depending on your metabolism and muscle movement in the treated area. Remember, there is minimal allergic or hypersensitivity risk with both Restylane® and Perlane®.

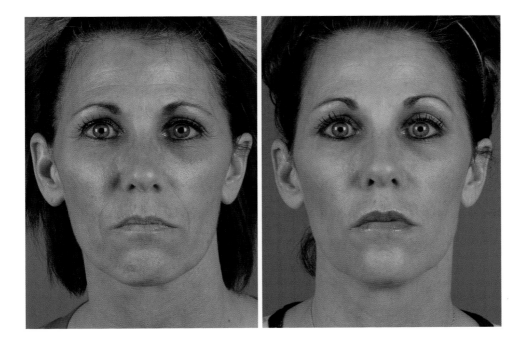

Patient had a combination of fillers and Botox® which reshaped her entire face. Note how the before picture shows signs of volume loss in the absence of sagging, making her an ideal candidate for this treatment.

2. *Juvéderm®*—another excellent hyaluronic acid filler. Due to its water-solubility, Juvéderm® is a softer filler and is therefore ideal for areas that see more muscle movement, such as the lips and the corners of the mouth. Juvéderm® can last more than six months, depending on the patient's metabolism. It is injected only for correction and causes tissue to become fuller over time. Like Restylane® and Perlane®, Juvéderm® is also reversible with hyaluronidase (an enzyme that breaks down hyaluronic acid).

3. *Voluma®*—another excellent higher density volumizing hyaluronic acid filler specifically indicated for use in enhancing the cheek (malar) area. It lasts a year or longer.

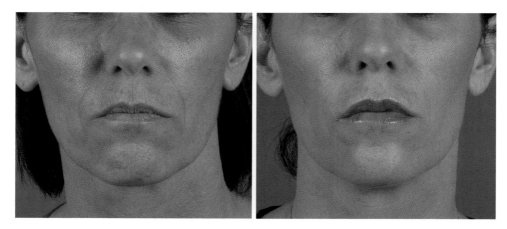

**Use of Juvederm® (hyaluronic acid filler) improved volume to the lips
and diminished lines around the mouth area**

4. *Belotero®*—a hyaluronic acid filler ideal for more superficial dermal filling. It works well on laugh and smile lines, especially around the mouth. It is also reversible. Its longevity is in the three to six month range.

5. *Radiesse®*—is used as a volumizing filler. It is primarily used for filling the cheek areas and if a patient has deep nasolabial folds. It is not used for lips, eyelids, tear troughs, or nose. It is made from hydroxyapatite, which is made from sea coral. Radiesse® is **not reversible** but does absorb over a twelve-to-eighteen-month period, so its effects are not permanent.

6. *Sculptra®*—is also a volumizer that gives you great results over time. It is gradual and requires two to four injection sessions spread over a three to four week period. It is made from a poly-L-lactic acid and helps replace lost collagen, especially in the cheek areas. Sculptra® is **not reversible** but does absorb over an eighteen to twenty-four month period, so its effects are not permanent.

You have probably heard of Botox®, but you may not know what it is. You are not alone. Botox® is not a filler, but like fillers, it is used to soften wrinkles as well as to smooth out the furrow in the brow and frown lines.

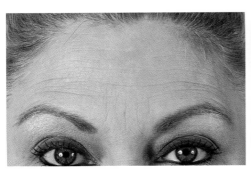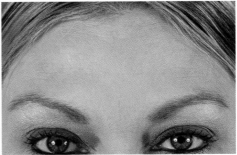

Botox® (onabotulinumtoxinA) was used to improve forehead wrinkles, furrow lines, and eyebrow shape

Botox® (onabotulinumtoxinA) is a brand name of a neuromodulator and is a well-recognized consumer word. **When we use the word Botox® throughout the book, we use it in a general manner to refer to all other neuromodulators including Xeomin® (incobotulinumtoxinA) and Dysport® (abobotulinumtoxinA). They are all excellent FDA-aproved neuromodulators.**

Botox® is a botulinum toxin type A FDA-approved neuromodulator in the same class as Xeomin® and Dysport®, which all work by temporarily weakening the muscles. This effect lasts about three to four months. Botox® was first used to treat problems with the eye muscles, spasms, and tics over forty years ago. Doctors noted a valuable side effect—patients had fewer wrinkles in the skin overlying the treated muscles because of the reduction in movement. Its usage for cosmetic purposes grew, making it a popular and attractive alternative or complement to fillers.

Botox® has been FDA-approved since 2002 to cosmetically soften wrinkles between the eyebrows. It can also be used "off-label" in many other areas of the face and body. **(Off-label use simply means that the FDA has not yet approved that particular drug, substance, or device for a certain area, indication, dosage, or population group. It does not mean it is illegal or unsafe. The FDA can't tell doctors how to prescribe the medicines they employ as long as they are approved for human use and the patient is told that it is an off-label use.)**

Fat Transfers—Using Your Own Fat as a Filler

One of the hottest topics at national and international medical symposiums on plastic surgery fell into one category—*FAT.* Fat transfers have taken on a growing importance in facial rejuvenation and modern body contouring. Fat makes a wonderful natural filler for the face. In some specific instances, it works well for augmenting breasts and/or buttocks either alone or with implants to create a more natural look.

Fat transfers have made a tremendous difference in facial rejuvenation, as the first sign of aging is loss of facial fat in the central face areas. Injections of fat into the deep malar (cheek areas) compartments of the face, along with other fat compartments, addresses this issue in a way that facelifts alone do not. This was accomplished by groundbreaking anatomic research done by us at UT Southwestern.

Note the major fat compartments in the image where I routinely inject fat for patients considering facial rejuvenation with or without a facelift.

Fat transfers carry a very low risk of allergic reaction because the fat is taken from your very own body. Fat transfers have revolutionized facial rejuvenation by bringing us the **"Lift and Fill" facelift** (see Chapter 6). Patients frequently opt to use fat transfers when they are having a facelift surgery. The advantage of this is that fat looks more natural than fillers in many areas of the face and lasts longer. The tradeoff is that the procedure must be done in the operating room or in a sterile procedure room. By contrast, soft tissue fillers can be used off the shelf, the procedure is far easier, and it can be done in an exam room of your surgeon's office. Recovery is also shorter. Both methods are viable and weighing the tradeoffs really comes down to your individual needs.

It is important that you understand the concepts and the science behind what makes good facial rejuvenation.

Loss of facial fat in the cheek and lower eye area is what causes that sunken look we all associate with aging. The use of your own fat to re-augment these areas can result in a more natural look than fillers. Once you have observed significant volume loss that has resulted in sagging, it may be time for a "Lift and Fill" facial rejuvenation using one's own fat.

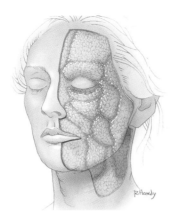
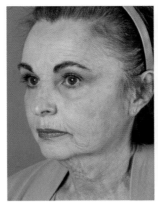
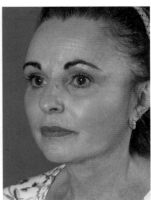

preoperative   postoperative

Fat transfers have revolutionized plastic surgery in total facial reju-venation where fat transfers are combined with a facelift (see above patient). **Gone are the days of the tight, pulled facelift.** Thankfully, we have entered into a time of the **"Lift and Fill" facial rejuvenation**, which provides natural- looking results because the technique is based upon the latest scientific findings of facial aging. **Just as fillers fill but don't lift, facelifts alone lift but do not fill! Lifting without filling can create an unnatural, pulled look that you want to avoid.**

The key here is to understand whether you need to lift, fill, or both. If you are experiencing only loss of volume, you may choose to have fat transfers. However, if you are experiencing sagging, you may benefit from a "Lift and Fill" facelift, which you'll discover in the next chapter.

Five Key Points to Remember:

1. Fillers fill, but do not lift. If you are experiencing significant facial sagging, see Chapter 6 for information on complete facial rejuvenation including the revolutionary "Lift and Fill" facelift.

2. Soft tissue fillers like Restylane®, Perlane®, Juvéderm®, Belotero®, and Voluma® are hyaluronic acid based and are reversible. Do not overdo or overuse them. Volumizers like Radiesse® and Sculptra® are used deep in the cheek area for volumizing and filling when you have lost significant volume. They are not reversible but are not permanent and last anywhere from eighteen to twenty-four months.

3. Botox® and other FDA-approved neuromodulators (Dysport® and Xeomin®) soften wrinkles and lines and can lift the eyebrows, but are not fillers.

4. Fat (your own) is an excellent filler, but more labor-intensive and has to be done in a procedure room or operating room. It is best when injected into deep compartments, not superficially, and will last longer than fillers.

5. It is imperative that you select an expert injector who understands facial aging, from one of the core four cosmetic medical specialties (see Chapter 3). Fillers, Botox®, and surgical facial rejuvenation have different indications, and your expert injector and you must understand what is needed when, why, and where for optimizing your facial rejuvenation.

Beyond the Facelift:

Your Options for Facial Rejuvenation

6

A patient recently told me the face staring back at her in the mirror wasn't someone she recognized. "My face looks tired and people at work ask me if I've been up all night."

She was still in her prime, yet her aging face no longer matched the youthful and vigorous way she felt. She is a successful executive at a Fortune 500 company, and felt she needed to look younger just to stay competitive in today's workplace. Whatever drives you to consider achieving a more youthful face, plastic surgery may help. In this chapter, we'll explore your options.

The Facial Rejuvenation Mirror Test

How do you know whether facial rejuvenation is right for you? Take this additional "Mirror Test." Stand in front of a mirror and ask yourself if any of these things bother you:

- Are your brows and eyelids droopy?
- Are your cheeks hollow or sagging—or both? Do you have jowls?
- Is your neck full and sagging? Are there marks and lines?
- Are your earlobes long, saggy, or deflated?
- Is your nose drooping?
- Are your lips deflated? Sagging? Full of wrinkles? Do you have laugh lines?

If you answered yes to any of these questions, and particularly if you answered yes to at least three, you may be a candidate for facial rejuvenation.

What Is Facial Rejuvenation and When Do You Need It?

Complete facial rejuvenation means improving the eyes, face, and neck. Patients typically inquire about "refreshing" their eyes first. This procedure usually precedes a face/neck lift.

The brows and the eyelids are the keys to the soul of an aging face. The eyelids age early and show the most telling changes, affected by gravity, sun, and poor sleep. Many people have baggy eyelids as well as general sagging and hollowing. **The important factor is keeping balance around the eyes—upper and lower. The goal is to look rested and more youthful. There has to be a blend of the eyelids and brows carefully with the cheeks and face for a balanced look.** The goal is to restore the eyelid, restore the eyelid/cheek junction, and remove the extra skin as needed. Also, lasers or peels can address wrinkling around the eyes.

For eye surgery, it may take four to six weeks for the incision scars to begin to soften and fade.

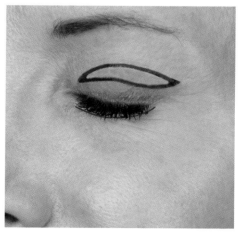

Incisions for upper and lower eyelid surgery

If you have brow sagging and extra upper eyelid skin, you are a candidate for both a browlift and an eyelift.

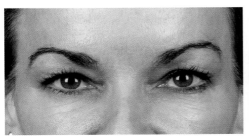
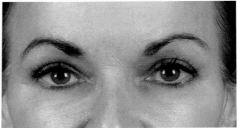

Natural appearing eyes after upper and lower eyelid rejuvenation

There are three types of browlifts:

1. **Endoscopic Browlift**—For minimal brow sagging, this is the least invasive with multiple, small incisions in the hairline.

2. **Temporal Browlift**—This is for patients with deeper furrows and outer brow sagging and uses slightly longer incisions than endoscopic, which allows repositioning of the outer brow.

3. **Coronal Browlift**—The incision is in the scalp from ear to ear lifting and removing excess skin. It is the most invasive of the three and requires more recovery time. The incision is usually hidden in the hair, unless the forehead needs to be shortened, in which case the incisions will be at the hairline.

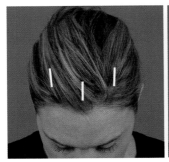
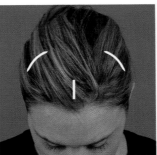
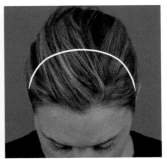

Endoscopic browlift   Temporal browlift   Coronal browlift

Once your eyelids and brows are addressed, you may want to consider rejuvenation of your face and neck. In prior decades, a facelift, also known as a rhytidectomy, was the answer to facial skin sagging. Unfortunately, these facelifts often resulted in an unnatural, pulled look. Even just ten years ago, plastic surgeons did not fully understand the role fat loss played in facial aging. It was, and still is, common practice to treat sagging simply by lifting the skin. On the surface, this makes sense—if you notice sagging, you want to lift and tighten the skin. **Yet the approach fails to address the true underlying reason for the sagging, which is loss of deep fat in the face. Lifting the skin without filling the face invariably results in the skin being over-tightened. Modern facial rejuvenation avoids this outcome by restoring fat in these compartments.**

Due to the ongoing, groundbreaking research on facial aging con-

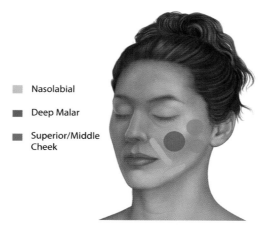

Nasolabial

Deep Malar

Superior/Middle Cheek

Four major fat compartments refilled with a "Lift and Fill" facelift

ducted at medical research centers, including the University of Texas Southwestern Medical Center where I practice, we now know far more about the science of aging. We know that most early facial sagging is the result of loss of malar (cheek) fat—the facial fat sitting just beneath the surface of the skin in the deep pockets below the eyes and in the cheeks. We have discovered the predictable patterns in which we lose fat from the face as we age. These realizations have revolutionized our approach to facelift surgery.

We now address the underlying loss of fat through fat transfers *in combination with* a facelift; we can literally **R**efresh, **R**eshape, and **R**ejuvenate your face, allowing a natural, youthful appearance with definition and tone. **This type of "Lift and Fill" facelift procedure can last ten years or more.**

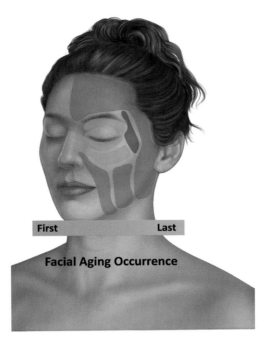

First   **Last**

Facial Aging Occurrence

Atrophy (loss) in the various fat compartments follows a predictable pattern over time. Eyelids and central cheek area age faster than other areas.

Fat transfers involve transferring fat from another part of the body to the face. Autologous fat (fat from your own body) is usually taken from the inner thigh and/or abdominal areas, as the fat cells are similar to the malar fat deposits in the face. Fat from your body minimizes the risk of allergic reaction or rejection.

As we have discussed, fillers can also be used to restore volume to the face. Generally, fillers work best for patients experiencing only a minor loss of fat. As patients continue to lose facial fat, substantial sagging begins. Once this starts, a more comprehensive facial rejuvenation is generally in order, no matter how old you are. This is the time you may want to consider rejuvenation techniques, which will not only fill but also lift. Such techniques specifically address sagging issues in the mid-face, lower-face, and neck areas.

Fillers definitely have their place in this process (see Chapter 5). Unfortunately, there are practitioners who do not fully understand the science of the aging of the human face. They often make the mistake of pushing fillers far too long into the aging process and in inappropriate amounts, believing that fillers will somehow "Lift *and* Fill."

A patient, Catherine, came to see me about this exact problem. She had so much filler added to her face, cheeks, and lips, she felt she now looked, in her own words, like an "overfilled marshmallow!" The good thing was that her fillers were hyaluronic acid, which can be reversed, and I did so with hyaluronidase in several sessions in my office. If other fillers such as Radiesse® and Sculptra® (great for volumizing) are used, they are not reversible. However, these fillers dissipate over a twelve-to-eighteen-month period.

So where did Catherine go wrong? Did she have a true filler expert and someone who really understood facial aging? Probably not. If she had taken the time to do the research, all the suffering and added expense could have been avoided! She chose the wrong doctor. Not a plastic surgeon. Not a dermatologist. Not a facial plastic surgeon. Not an oculoplastic surgeon. Instead, she went to a family doctor with no expertise or experience with fillers. Unfortunately, Catherine had someone pumping too many fillers, when she really needed complete facial rejuvenation. While fillers may seem more convenient or a quick fix, you need a true facial aging expert surgeon that knows when it is time for surgery versus just using fillers.

Although fillers are great, they are often overused. When one begins to lose facial fat and sagging begins, fillers alone are no longer the answer. You want to pick a surgeon that understands the science of aging. This way you can be sure that he or she has the know-how and expertise to provide you with a custom-tailored treatment plan that you need and deserve.

Ask for Before-and-After Photos!

We highly recommend asking to see before-and-after photos of a surgeon's previous patients. Also, you need to see more than one set of photos. Make sure the "after" photos were taken at least one year post-op. **The after photos should look younger and better, but not different. They should look exceptionally improved.**

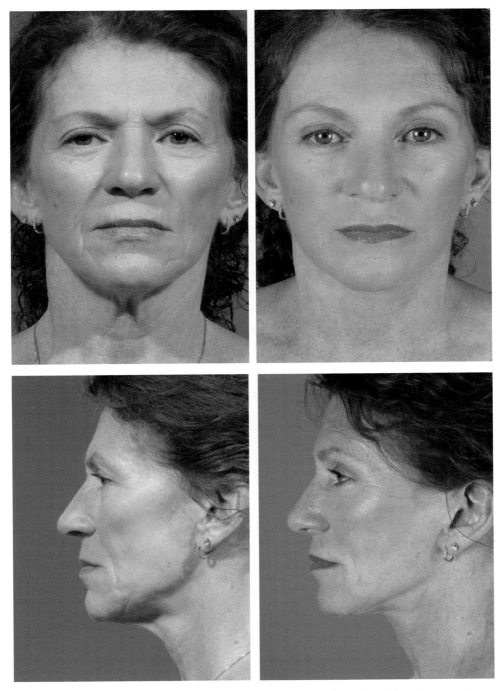

Natural rejuvenation in this patient with complete facial rejuvenation ("Lift and Fill" face/neck lift, endotemporal browlift, upper and lower eyelids, fat compartment augmentation, and perioral laserbrasion)

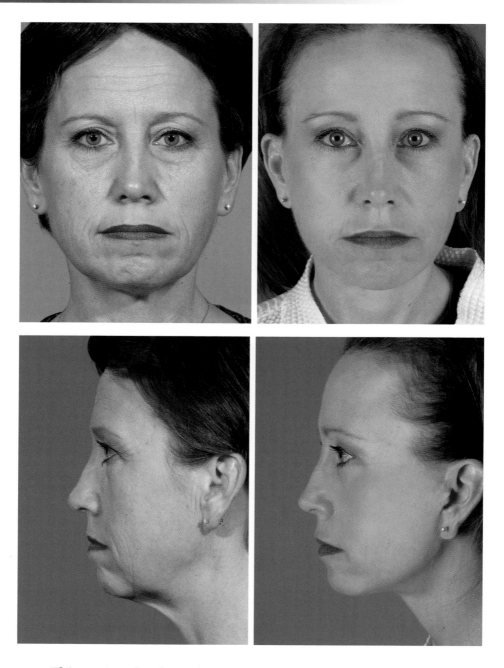

This patient has benefited from modern "Lift and Fill" facial rejuvenation techniques resulting in a natural, youthful appearance. Note the patient's sagging was corrected *without* pulling the skin tight. Thanks to the redistribution and addition of fat, this patient looks natural and younger and no one would know she had surgery.

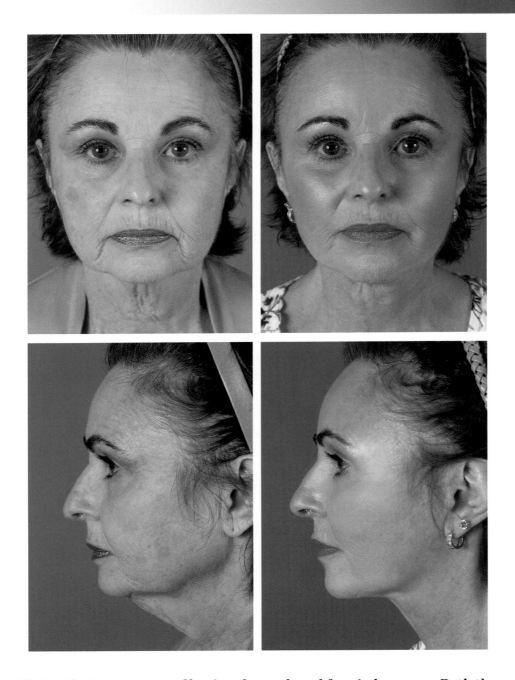

Notice the importance of having the neck and face in harmony. Both the neck itself and the face as a whole are much improved.

Don't Underestimate the Importance of the Neck in Facial Harmony

One of the most common complaints I hear from unhappy patients is about their sagging necks. **To make a complete facial rejuvenation, one must address and correct the neck and face *together* for overall harmony. It is important to pay attention to the alignment and appearance of individual features and the face as a whole.** You cannot do a spot-by-spot facial rejuvenation—it takes a surgeon with an eye for overall balance.

Are You Physically and Emotionally Prepared?

As with any elective medical procedure, you should only undergo facial rejuvenation when you are in good health—both physically and mentally. ***When making this decision, you want your body and immune system rested and in good shape in order to minimize the risk of complications. Facial rejuvenation is not advisable if you have significant underlying medical issues.***

Furthermore, you want to be sure you are having elective surgery for the right reasons and making decisions with a clear mind and discerning eye. There are many things you can do to make changes in your life. Depression, for example, may cause a skewed body image, which may lead to unnecessary aesthetic surgery.

Commonly Asked Questions About Facial Rejuvenation

If you have been intrigued about the possibilities of modern facial rejuvenation, but still have questions, you're not alone. In the second half of this chapter, we'll answer the most common—and essential—questions about navigating your appearance.

What Is the Recovery Time and Process for Facial Rejuvenation?

Recovery times vary, so ask your surgeon what to expect, and keep the lines of communication open throughout your recovery. Don't hesitate to ask questions, no matter the subject or concern.

After your procedure, your surgeon will apply head dressings and/or bandages in order to protect your face during your post-op recovery. I then transfer my patients to a peaceful recovery area where they may remain for approximately two days. This will vary from surgeon to surgeon. My patients stay in one of our around-the-clock-staffed nursing care facilities, in ambulatory settings at both UT Southwestern Medical Center and at our Northpark offices in Dallas. This is for their safety and convenience, and allows their surgical companion to supply the best possible care.

During this rest time, sleep elevated at a 40 to 45 degree angle to avoid swelling. You will experience some drainage in the first few days, which is completely normal. Do not pull on or tamper with any surgical drains or dressings. If you feel there is an issue, consult your surgeon or your surgeon's medical staff. Have your surgical companion with you at these early post-op times.

The first day after surgery, you will be put on a light diet. In most cases, head dressings and drains will be removed on the second day. I allow my facial rejuvenation patients to shower after the dressings and drains are removed. Your hair will be washed for you before you go home. Short, intermittent walks will help you with circulation and relax the body.

Virtually all patients will experience some degree of bruising in the lower face and neck areas—this is standard and part of the healing process. These will show up in the first 48 hours and gradually diminish for most patients within a week to ten days.

Ask your surgeon when you can return to eating normally and make sure you know the specifics about returning to exercise and other aspects of daily life. Do not exercise for three to four weeks, and especially avoid swimming.

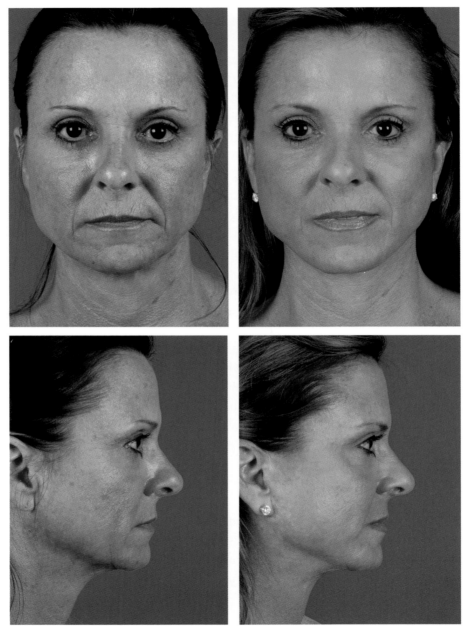

Patient with "Lift and Fill" facelift, TCA peel central face, and laser around the mouth

Will I Experience Discomfort After My Facial Surgery?

You may be prescribed an antianxiety medication, such as Valium® or Xanax®. If you cannot take certain drugs, such as tranquilizers or pain medications, discuss this with your surgeon beforehand. Inform your surgeon of other medications you are taking and any drug allergies you may have.

There should be little to no pain during recovery, as the medical staff will administer helpful medications. Any significant lasting discomfort may signal a deeper issue, as facelifts in general do not create much pain. Any serious pain or discomfort should be reported to your surgeon.

Numbness in the cheek and neck area is entirely normal and can last up to a year, but will go away with time. With facial rejuvenation, you can expect to have a gentle and gradual recovery period of about two to three weeks. You will probably make much progress in the first five to seven days, but this will vary depending upon your procedure or procedures. If facial rejuvenation is done in conjunction with a laser or chemical peel, there will be approximately seven additional days of recuperation necessary to allow for the skin surface to fully heal, for a total of approximately three weeks of recovery time.

In my experience, there was very little to no discomfort to the face, but the sutures were slightly uncomfortable as they tightened with healing. It was by no means unbearable. I found the healing process to be pretty much what I had expected after doing my research. Just being prepared and knowing what to expect made a real difference and kept me calm.

As after any surgical procedure, go easy on yourself and follow your surgeon's instructions. You may feel somewhat uncomfortable, but remember that it is all very temporary. Focus on the results and let your body recover without putting time limits on yourself.

If you have deeper concerns or experience a significant amount of pain, always consult your surgeon, who will keep your safety and comfort in mind. In the meantime, relax and rest. Through this process, you will learn a lot about the way your body works and takes care of itself. Everyone heals differently, but the basics of recovery are essentially the

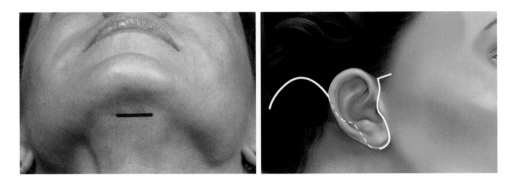

Incisions are concealed in natural folds

same for most people. Have faith in how you will heal and trust in your surgeon—you will soon recover.

Where Will My Incisions Be and Will They Be Noticeable?

The placement of incisions can vary depending on the specifics of your procedure. They are generally placed within the hairline and natural contours of the face and around the ears. There may be modified shorter incisions around the ears, depending on the specifics of your procedure. This provides maximum concealment.

Having a trusted plastic surgery expert makes a significant difference in the appearance of your facelift and neck lift incisions. They should be mostly unnoticeable and hard to see within ten to twelve weeks. As months go by, they will gradually fade and eventually should be almost undetectable.

One of my closest friends saw five different plastic surgeons over the years regarding lower facial rejuvenation. She was very scared about looking different and having noticeable incision scars. Even after doing her homework, she had these same fears. What put her at ease was seeing me in person—she was amazed. I didn't look different, just "better," as she put it, and she couldn't find my incision scars on her own. She made an appointment with Dr. Rohrich and immediately developed the rapport and trust she was seeking. Her procedure went great and the outcome was an even better, more youthful her. She is happy, and, in case you are wondering, her scars have almost entirely faded!

When Will I Look Normal to Others?

Most people begin to look fully natural in about three to four weeks, but everyone heals differently. By that time, it will be less apparent to people that you have undergone a procedure. All they will see is the rested, refreshed, new you. People will only know you had work done if you choose to tell them!

Avoid aspirin, Advil, and fish oil supplements for at least two weeks pre- and post-op, because they will change the course of your recovery by increasing bruising. Makeup can disguise small scars or redness and bruising. By four to six weeks, most of the major swelling will be gone. It may take up to six months for you to consider your recovery to be complete.

How Long Will a Facelift Last?

A correctly performed facelift normally lasts up to ten years or longer, depending upon your genetics, what type of facelift you receive, and how well you maintain your results.

Naturally, you will continue to age after your facelift—fat volume will naturally decrease and skin will further sag. So while a facelift has some permanent *effects*, it is not a permanent *solution*. That is why lifelong maintenance is so important to maintain your result and youthful face (see Chapter 13 for more information).

You may eventually want to look into additional procedures, particularly if you did not have total facial rejuvenation all at one time. If you experience further sagging and fat loss, you might consider touchup fillers or even another facelift in approximately ten years. Again, we stress the importance of preventative care and maintenance. Talk with your plastic surgeon about your skin—know how it changes and ages, and find ways to set yourself up for success.

Self-care and long-term maintenance are essential. For the most part, these are the things you should already be doing to take care of your face and prevent further aging. Protect yourself against UV damage, stay hydrated, and minimize the stress in your life. Simple tactics, like a good skin care regimen and applying sunscreen will minimize the need for a facelift, maximize the benefits of one, and prolong its positive effects.

You will also want to be careful with putting on weight after a facelift, as this can alter the overall composition of your face.

What a Facelift Won't Do

A facelift is rejuvenation surgery intended to improve your appearance; it's not the creation of a brand-new face! Being realistic is vital. A good facelift can take off about ten to fifteen years maximum. I have worked in this field for over twenty-five years and not once have I seen anyone in his or her sixties who could pass for twenty, no matter how much work they have had done. Make no mistake—there is a point of diminishing return where too much work will make you look worse, not better!

Ancillary Procedures to Facial Rejuvenation

Now let's look at procedures that complement a "Lift and Fill" facelift. You will need a surgeon who is well versed in the science of aging and can help craft a comprehensive total facial rejuvenation plan that meets your individual needs.

Although these procedures do not have to be performed at the same time as your facial rejuvenation, doing so has certain advantages. Since they target the same general area of the body (your face and neck), performing them simultaneously will allow your surgeon to balance your facial features. Second, this has the added benefit of decreasing your recovery time and lets you heal from all the treatments at once.

Ancillaries help minimize the contrast between your newly rejuvenated mid/lower face and the rest of your face and neck. For example, a facelift coupled with fat transfers will reduce or soften wrinkles in your cheeks, but will have no effect on the wrinkles around your eyes and mouth. This might leave a notable contrast in the appearance of skin across your face. For this reason, it is a good idea to address the whole face at once with a complete, thoroughly inclusive treatment plan.

Here are some of the other procedures you may want to consider:

- **Lasers and Peels:** These target the wrinkles that a facelift will not remove, especially those wrinkles around your lips and eyes. Understandably, combining procedures will change the amount of needed recovery time.

- **Earlobe Rejuvenation:** The earlobes lose volume as we age, causing them to appear thin and flat, and may lengthen or droop. Lobes that have lost volume can be rejuvenated with injections of autologous fat (fat from your own body) or a filler. I use hyaluronic acid fillers that can last for about a year or longer. If thinning earlobes have led to elongated earlobes, your surgeon can repair these during your facial rejuvenation. This is a telltale sign of facial aging, and I prefer to always correct earlobes along with a facelift in order to achieve greater facial harmony.

- **Chin Implant:** While a facelift will reduce sagging skin and thereby reduce the appearance of a double chin, the procedure will not change the overall structure of the area. To achieve an improved effect, a chin implant is often added in conjunction with a facelift or rhinoplasty. You may be a good candidate for a chin implant if you have a weak chin but a normally functioning jaw.

- **Upper Lip Shortening:** The upper lip thins and lengthens with age, which is also correctable by making a small incision just below the nose to shorten and turn the lip slightly up. One of my patients told me that this one simple procedure had the greatest effect on making her look young again.

Complementary procedures are great because they emphasize facial balance and harmony. Skillfully combining treatments and procedures can result in a sum that is greater than its parts. You want a surgeon that is not going to change your appearance, but make you a better and younger looking you. Talk to your surgeon about your wishes, and together you can work out a comprehensive long-term plan for your total facial restoration.

Five Key Points to Remember:

1. Facial rejuvenation is indicated for patients experiencing facial sagging—this is when fillers alone are no longer enough. Facial aging is primarily due to fat loss.

2. Modern facial rejuvenation demands both a "Lift and Fill" face/neck lift to combat the loss of facial fat and give a long-lasting natural result. Fat transfer using autologous fat (one's own fat) during facial rejuvenation achieves optimal results.

3. Share your top three concerns you have selected using the Mirror Test with your plastic surgeon. Work with your surgeon to develop a plan of what you want corrected.

4. The goal of facial rejuvenation is to enhance, not change your appearance—you want to look like you, only better and younger. This means you need to have your brow, face, and neck in proportion.

5. Maintain your results by continuing to practice great skin care as outlined in Chapter 4.

The Nose Knows:

Why Rhinoplasty Is So Challenging

7

A patient of mine, Georgia, came to see me three months after her rhinoplasty. She wanted to let me know how her surgery had changed her life. She suddenly felt taken more seriously at work. People had begun to notice her at the gym and on the street—she could see them giving approving second looks. Before, she had a long nose with a pronounced hump that she never liked.

"It's the best thing I ever did for myself," she said. "I have never felt so confident!"

This kind of feedback affirms the value of plastic surgery. There's nothing more satisfying for me, as a doctor and a plastic surgeon, than to see a patient so appreciative and transformed. My patients often experience an improved sense of well-being.

Rhinoplasty is especially prone to induce these feelings because the nose is such a central and prominent feature that acts as an anchor for the whole face—providing facial balance and harmony. Many rhinoplasty patients have considered the procedure for some time. They may be dissatisfied with a specific aspect of their nose: maybe it is too large, too small, strangely shaped, has small humps or is asymmetrical. Others see nothing technically "wrong" with their nose, but simply want a nose shape and size that better matches their facial features.

The nose's "central" role in facial harmony means that minor imperfections can have exaggerated effects on the rest of your appearance. Fortunately, it also means that minor surgical changes can have dramatically positive effects. Careful attention must be taken when working with noses. As an art, it is a matter of millimeters and experience, with little to no margin for error. You need a true expert to do your rhinoplasty, so please review the information in Chapter 3. (The ***Three Magic Questions***.)

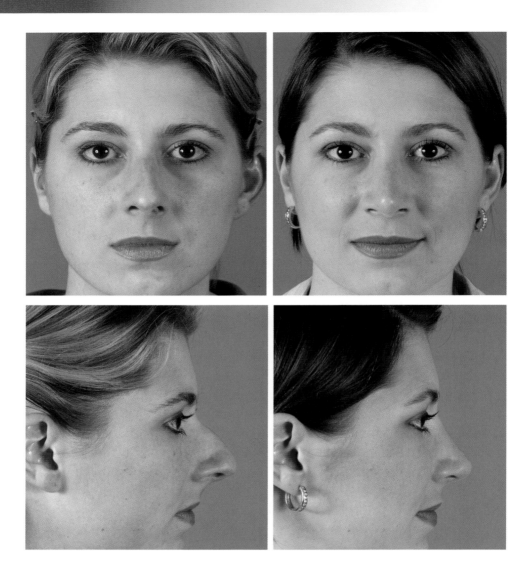

This patient wanted to have her nose match her face. She did not like her long nose and the large hump. Note how her new nose looks natural and improves her overall facial balance.

The level of finesse required for rhinoplasty involves considerable proficiency and experience. When it comes to your nose, it's essential to try to get it right the first time. Unfortunately, the most "informed" rhinoplasty patients only take the time to educate themselves after a first surgery has been unsuccessful.

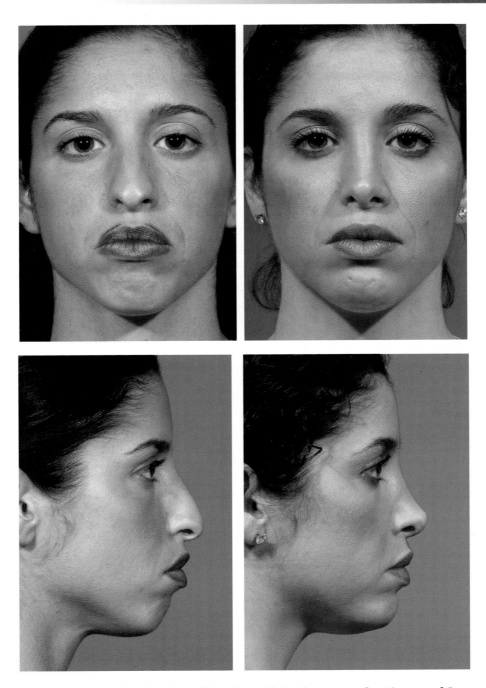

This patient desired a refined nasal tip, hump reduction, and I suggested the chin implant. You can see how greatly improved her facial balance is post-op with her new nose and chin.

To start, we want you to again take the Mirror Test: list the top three things that cause you concern regarding your nose. Make a long and candid observation and try to identify what specifically you want to change. Prioritize your thoughts on paper.

The list below is by no means comprehensive, but represents many of the most aesthetic revisions that are made to the nose:

> - Altering/reshaping of the nasal bridge (removing the bump)
>
> - Reducing the width of the nose (too wide when I smile)
>
> - Correcting the shape of the nose (too big or too small)
>
> - Reshaping the nasal tip (too wide or asymmetrical)
>
> - Reducing the size of the nostrils (flares when you talk)
>
> - Correcting the angle between the nose and upper lip (too long or too short)

Due to the complexity and difficulty of rhinoplasty procedures, three changes are generally a healthy maximum to attempt during a single procedure. Take this list to your consultation so you can work with your surgeon to develop a realistic plan for reaching your surgery goals.

A patient came to me with a list of ten things about her nose that she wanted fixed. I appreciated her candor, but the results she wanted were unrealistic and would not have matched her face. During consultation, it became clear that it was only her nasal hump and bulbous tip she wanted fixed. I showed the proposed changes on a computer image and she loved them. She did very well and is still delighted with her nose several years post-op.

The lesson here is important—you have to be honest and realistic about what a rhinoplasty can and cannot do for you. If you and your surgeon cannot come to terms on this important issue, don't have the surgery or seek another opinion.

The Power of Saying No!

A European woman visited my office for a rhinoplasty consultation. She wanted only a large hump removed and adamantly refused other work that would be needed to preserve or improve her facial harmony. I imaged her nose to show that only removal of the hump on a long wide nose with a bulbous (round) nasal tip would leave her with a large nose and a disproportionate end result. She refused to listen, and I ultimately declined to perform the procedure. This may sound harsh, but I will not operate on someone willing to put their face and nose out of aesthetic harmony. The lesson here is clear—when you find your true rhinoplasty expert, please listen to his or her opinion and make sure it matches your top three goals.

Computer imaging is a great educational tool that I use to show patients how they may look post-op. Not infrequetly with rhinoplasty, your surgeon may suggest a chin implant if you have a small chin. Don't think of it as "upselling" as this may help achieve improved nasal and facial balance.

If you learn anything here, learn from us how to find your personal best rhinoplasty expert. Be cautious about accepting surgical advice and input from friends and family. They might attempt to dissuade you from surgery and you may hear pessimistic messages. Keep in mind that these are only opinions, and ultimately, you must make this decision for yourself. I recommend that you focus your research on facts first and not opinions. Trust the knowledge of your surgeon and follow your own heart.

Not All Rhinoplasty Is Strictly Aesthetic

Many people seek nose surgery for reasons unrelated to aesthetics. Patients who have suffered nasal-related congenital deformities or

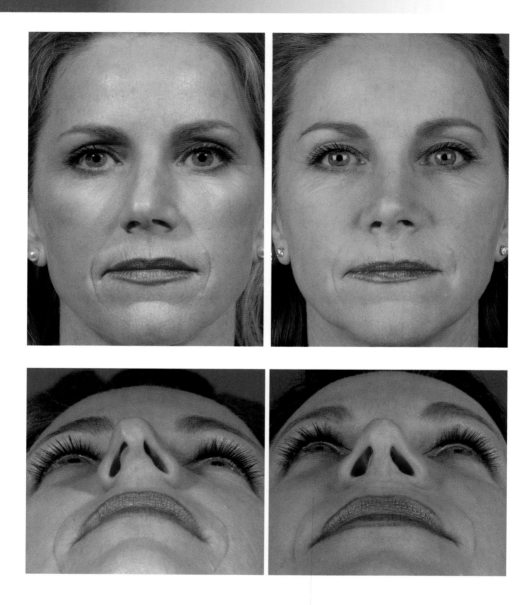

Patient who had a deviated septum corrected which greatly improved her function and cosmetic appearance

sustained physical trauma are prime candidates for rhinoplasty. A broken nose resulting in an altered shape or function can be corrected with surgery.

A deviated septum can be due to trauma or perhaps the person was born that way. This condition can create difficulties with breathing, induce snoring or sleep apnea, lead to sinus infections, and cause a host of other medical problems. A true rhinoplasty expert can and will, in one procedure, repair both the inside of your nose and make the outside look great as well. As an added potential benefit, your insurance company may cover inside (functional aspect) rhinoplasty work. Check with your doctor's office about this.

When Is a Secondary Surgery Necessary?

Even with a true rhinoplasty expert, you may need a revision after a year or longer due to wound healing problems. The most common reasons for performing a revision nasal surgery are excess scar formation post-rhinoplasty or loss of nasal support. This cannot be controlled or anticipated, as it depends on how the body heals and how you respond to surgery. I talk openly and honestly about what I can and cannot do. If there should be a need for a minor revision, it can usually be done in an office under local anesthesia. The most common modification or minor revision in my practice is to correct residual nasal fullness due to scar tissue. Most major revision rhinoplasty procedures need to be done at least twelve months post-op to allow for nasal wound healing.

Secondary (revision) rhinoplasty makes up about 50 percent of my rhinoplasty practice. Reworking another doctor's rhinoplasty is very challenging and often requires grafts from other parts of the body such as the ear or the rib cage. (See Chapter 10 on how to manage revision surgery.)

The Seven Point Checklist for Rhinoplasty Patients

In order to prepare you for surgery, we have compiled a seven point checklist of considerations so you can get the best care.

1. Choosing the Right Surgeon

Rhinoplasty requires a specialist. Therefore, look for a board certified plastic surgeon or otolaryngologist (ENT) with expertise and experience in rhinoplasty—these are the only two groups of surgeons who work in this area and have the specific training to be a true rhinoplasty expert.

Ask your prospective rhinoplasty surgeon how many nose surgeries they have performed. They should have recent and ongoing experience in the exact procedure you desire. Be sure to request before-and-after photos of other patients that demonstrate the changes you inquire about. Now is the time to bring up your top three concerns. Are they in harmony with what you want, and are you realistic about what can and cannot be done?

Do you have a true rhinoplasty expert? (Ask the **Three Magic Questions** from Chapter 3.) This is vital to getting the best possible result since rhinoplasty is the most challenging procedure in plastic surgery.

Before you decide on a surgeon, make sure you are absolutely comfortable with them, no hesitations. Dr. Rohrich gives his personal cell number to his patients and tells them to phone or text him at any time. I've not heard of many plastic surgeons or other doctors who do this. Take your time to find the right rhinoplasty surgeon for you, and do as much research as possible to become an informed patient/consumer.

Remember that no question is too "dumb," except for the one you don't ask. Be a proactive patient—this surgery is complicated and you do not want to hide anything from your surgeon.

2. Make Sure You Schedule Adequate Time Away From Work

Allow for seven to ten days of good recovery, possibly longer depending on how quickly your body heals. There will be swelling and bruising, though the amount varies for each patient. Your surgeon will apply an outer splint, and possibly an internal one, too, if you have inner-nose work done. This will be worn for about a week. After the nasal splint comes off, I usually apply light tape to the nose. Do not tamper with your dressings unless instructed by your surgeon and please follow the post-op instructions given to you.

3. What You Can Do to Reduce Bruising and Swelling

Typically, most of the initial swelling will occur in the first seven to ten days. Minor swelling will gradually diminish over several months to a year. The slight numbness you notice will usually go away within six months. You will know that the healing is finished when the softness returns to your nasal tip—twelve to fifteen months in most cases. It may take longer if you have thick skin, are male, or are having a revision rhinoplasty.

Keeping the nasal airways and nostrils clean and open after surgery will help you recover more comfortably and faster—your surgeon will show you how to do this. Be careful not to disturb the tissue and structures of your new nose as they heal. While bruising and swelling are unavoidable, there are things you can do to minimize their appearance and alleviate possible discomfort.

- Keep your head elevated. Apply cold compresses and ice gel packs to the eyes, changing them often in order to keep the area cool. I recommend 20 minutes on and 20 minutes off throughout the day. This helps immensely during the first week after surgery.

- Avoid aspirin, other anti-inflammatory medications, and fish oil supplements for up to two weeks before and after your surgery. These products act as blood thinners, which will exacerbate swelling and bruising. Your surgeon will provide you with alternative pain medications to use after surgery.

- Avoid wearing any glasses for three to four weeks. Glasses apply pressure to the bridge of the nose, which can cause indentations when worn shortly after surgery. Ask your surgeon to show you how to tape your glasses from the forehead so as to avoid putting pressure on your new nose. Contact lenses are fine after three to five days.

- There are many effective homeopathic remedies for bruising and swelling. Products containing arnica (an herb) and bromelain (a pineapple stem extract) are two commonly used natural products that can reduce swelling and bruising—both can be purchased over the counter.

4. Normal Post-Op Rhinoplasty: What to Expect After Surgery

Surgery, as a whole, can be stressful. You already know that there may be a certain degree of discomfort. Here are some other things you may experience after surgery:

- *Feeling congested*. Do not actively blow your nose for the first three to four weeks—this is very important. Speak to your surgeon as there are treatments to ease sinus congestion. An example is the use of a sterile saline spray six to eight times per day for six weeks post-op.

- *Swelling around the face and eyes*. This should subside within seven to ten days—speak with your surgeon if puffiness persists for longer. Swelling in the nose itself will linger for a time longer. This is normal.

- *Bleeding from the nostrils during the first several days.* Minor bleeding is typical; inform your surgeon immediately if you experience excessive bleeding. If you need to change your nasal drip pad more than once every 30 minutes post-op due to bright red bleeding, call your rhinoplasty surgeon.

- *Feelings of fatigue.* The stresses of planning and undergoing surgery can exact a considerable toll on your mind and body. Pain medications and the lingering effects of anesthesia can further tire you. Plan ahead and expect to take it

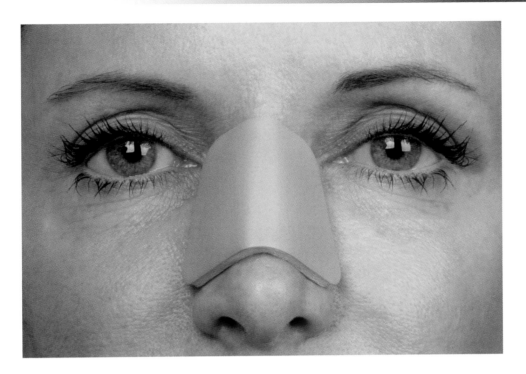

Nasal splint used after rhinoplasty

easy for a few weeks. Do not raise your heart rate to over 100 beats per minute for the first three weeks. You can typically resume full exercise by four weeks.

- *Impatience.* "Bouncing back" doesn't happen in a day. The swelling must diminish and the results mature before the nose can "be itself." Inflammation will fade over time. It is common to see an asymmetrical appearance to the nose right after surgery—don't be alarmed. As I tell my patients, I don't leave the operating room until your nose looks the best it can!

- *Dry, irritated inner nose and sinus passages.* The inner nose produces over a quart of moisture every day in order to keep tissues hydrated. This process is impeded by surgery. It is absolutely necessary to use an over-the-counter nasal saline spray, such as OCEAN® Spray (the nasal mist, not the fruit juice cocktail!), throughout the day for the first six to eight weeks.

- *It is NOT normal to run a fever (temperature above 101° F.) or to have chills, redness (that is not just bruising), or pus coming out of the nose.* These are rare occurrences, but they could be signs of infection and should be reported to your surgeon immediately.

As Dr. Rohrich states, all of these symptoms are normal—but only up to a point. Speak with your surgeon beforehand about what to expect and follow up if you have concerns. Remember this is a process. Rome wasn't built in a day—and neither are new noses!

5. What to Expect in the Post-Op Appointments

Your first post-op appointment will be scheduled approximately seven days after your surgery. At this point, any splints (external or internal) may likely be removed. The nasal sutures are also removed at this point.

After these items are removed, you will need a short period of readjustment and may feel a bit tired. You will need someone to drive you to and from the first post-op appointment.

When your splints come off, your recovery becomes very exciting! You will feel encouraged by the progress. The removal of a splint does not signal the end of healing—you must take great care to protect your new nose. Things will happen naturally, so there is no need to rush the process.

6. Easing Back Into Exercise—When and How Much?

At the minimum, you should wait at least three to four weeks, but always consult your surgeon. Avoid other strenuous types of activity, such as heavy lifting and yard work.

While you are healing, an elevated heart rate will increase blood flow and can possibly lead to excess swelling, bruising, and even bleeding.

Furthermore, you might give yourself a headache and suffer dizziness. Limit yourself to gentle walking for the time being.

*Focus on **initial** recovery as this may take three to four weeks and varies from person to person. In addition to limiting exercise, be sure to check with your surgeon on any travel plans or returning to work.*

7. When Will Recovery Be Over? The Final Outcome.

You will look mostly normal to yourself and others in four to six weeks, but it may take a year or more for your nose to settle into its final form. Typically, swelling reduces in stages over time. The worst swelling is experienced in the first week or two. The area around the nose will be the first to return to normal. After about four to six weeks, there will be another noticeable decrease in swelling, this time in the actual nose itself. At this point, only you will notice residual swelling. Getting past the first two weeks is a major first step in recovery. You will feel much better once the splints are off.

Most of your healing process will be determined by genetics. Resting and following post-op instructions are key in producing the desired outcome. The nose is considered recovered and normal once it has naturally softened, blends perfectly with the rest of the face, and has returned to full-feeling sensation. When your nasal tip no longer feels hard, then your healing will be complete.

Friends and patients whom I have talked with all had the same comment: "I am so congested!" My friends really had to make an effort not to blow their noses. They all said that congestion was the most notable part of recovery. Consult with your surgeon as you may be able to use a decongestant post-op.

It's also important to be patient with the swelling. With each passing day, the swelling will go down a bit more, you'll feel better, and you will be thrilled with the new you that smiles back in the mirror—it's just a matter of time!

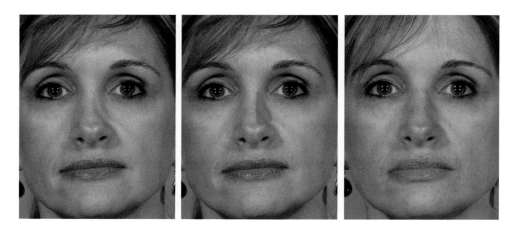

This patient had a previous rhinoplasty done by another surgeon with left mid-nose collapse that was corrected with Restylane® (a safe and soft hyaluronic acid filler). Post-injection at one year, she did not want any additional surgery and still looks excellent.

Liquid Non-Surgical Rhinoplasty and Does It Really Work?

A liquid rhinoplasty uses a filler (such as Restylane®) to augment or fill in an area of the nose so the patient can experience the nose he or she may want before having the real surgery. This is a temporary fix to improve nasal shape and contour the nose. It is also very useful to correct subtle **secondary nasal deformities that cannot be corrected by surgery**. Results can last about one year.

Five Key Points to Remember:

1. Rhinoplasty is the most difficult of all aesthetic plastic surgeries. Find the appropriate surgeon (either ENT facial plastic surgeon or plastic surgeon) with expertise in rhinoplasty. This is especially true for **secondary rhinoplasty**.

2. You will see the final results of your rhinoplasty after approximately one year. It may be longer if you have thick skin, are male, or are having revision rhinoplasty.

3. Keep your expectations realistic—address your top three concerns. Be in sync with your surgeon about what can, and more importantly *cannot,* be done to improve your nose.

4. A great rhinoplasty looks natural and balanced with overall facial harmony.

5. As with all plastic surgery, give yourself adequate time to heal before you return to your prior level of activity.

Breast Enhancements:

When to Do a Breast Lift, When to Do an Implant—And When Reconstruction is Needed

8

Popular culture tends to portray breast augmentation as the only kind of breast enhancement that exists. In reality, there are many breast surgical procedures for optimizing size, shape, comfort, and overall appearance of the breasts. In this chapter, we will explore these options and their benefits. We will focus on the four most common breast enhancement procedures:

1. *Breast Augmentation*—which uses an implant or the patient's own body tissue. The surgeon augments or fills the breasts in order to achieve increased breast volume and balance the chest with the rest of the body. This can be an inherited condition or due to body changes including hormone imbalances, menopause, aging, pregnancy, breastfeeding, or weight loss. Over 200,000 women in the United States have this common surgery every year.

2. *Breast Lift*—in which the surgeon lifts sagging breasts to treat ptosis (drooping). This is often done in conjunction with augmentation to remedy sagging breasts. A lift is often also performed in combination with a reduction.

3. *Breast Reduction*—reducing breasts that are too large. This brings the breasts into proportion with the rest of the body.

4. *Breast Reconstruction*—recreating the breast structure after a mastectomy to treat breast cancer.

A word of caution: Before undergoing breast augmentation, be sure that you know your risk for breast cancer. One in eight American women will be diagnosed with breast cancer during their lifetime. Breast implants are **not** known to cause cancer and will not interfere with accurate cancer screening, but you need to be reasonably sure that you are not at risk due to your family history.

Yearly mammograms are not generally indicated for those under the age of forty (as stated by the American Cancer Society guidelines), unless you have a history of breast cancer in your family (especially on your mother's side). Further important guidelines are regular self-examinations, as are clinical breast exams (CBE) by a health professional—at least every three years. After age forty, women should have a breast exam by a health professional every year. Know your family history and make certain you understand breast cancer prevention and care guidelines (visit www.cancer.org, the American Cancer Society website, for more information). We concur with these standards completely and promote breast care first and foremost in consideration with cosmetic surgery.

No matter the procedure, the primary goal is reshaping the breasts to create balance with the rest of the body. I discourage patients who have plans to over-enlarge their breasts, as the results appear obvious and unnatural, possibly even inducing side effects (including excessive scarring and breast sagging).

Breast enhancement is a process that requires total-body consideration to look proportionate and balanced. There is no "one perfect size"—your breasts should match your body shape and, above all, be comfortable for exercising and everyday life. As you can see, this is a very personal procedure, and the right plastic surgeon will be able to help you identify and achieve perfectly tailored results.

Breast Augmentation

With breast augmentation, you have four major areas to consider:

1. Placement of incisions and implant placement

2. Implant size/sizing

3. Type of implant

4. Risks

Incision and Implant Placement

To gain access to the inside of the breasts, your surgeon will make a few strategic incisions. The placement of the incisions balances ease of surgical access against scar visibility. Talk with your surgeon about your options and learn about the benefits and downsides of each type of incision.

The three most common incisions for breast augmentation are as follows:

1. *Inframammary Incision (under the breast fold)*—in my opinion, this is the best incision for most patients. The main advantage is that this method allows the surgeon a direct route to the inside of the breast, which increases the chances of correcting subtle breast asymmetries. The scars are usually hidden from view. Loss of nipple sensation is only 5 to 7 percent—the lowest rate of any incision type. In most but not all cases, numbness disappears over time. The same incision site can be used for removing and replacing implants later.

2. *Transaxillary Incision (in the armpit)*—has the advantage of hiding scars inside the armpits, away from the breast area. It also makes the operation more complicated and results in a higher revision rate because it is so far from direct breast tissue. The armpit incision is not likely to provide total scar concealment and most of my patients find that there is little, if any, real visibility

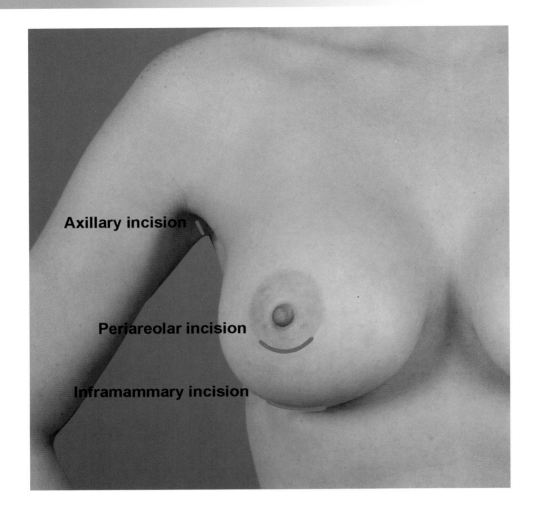

Axillary incision

Periareolar incision

Inframammary incision

Common incisions for a breast augmentation

advantage over an inframammary incision. The loss of nipple sensation is about 10 percent with this approach, and, in some cases, can cause numbness in the inner arm area.

3. ***Periareolar Incision*** *(around the nipple)*—attempts to hide the scar within and around the lower areola. While the color and texture between the areola and the breast skin can help conceal the scar, there is slightly higher risk for loss of nipple sensation (10 to 15 percent). I rarely use this approach because it results in increased risk of bacteria reaching the implant.

I almost exclusively use the inframammary incision unless there is a specific reason to do otherwise. This incision provides optimal direct access and the least chance of complication in my experience. There are surgeons who work exclusively with one kind of approach. For example, if you are set on having a transaxillary (in the armpit) incision, seek out an expert breast plastic surgeon who specializes in this technique.

Where Is the Implant Placed?

Breast augmentation normally involves the insertion of an implant beneath the breast tissue (subglandular) or under the pectoralis muscle (subpectoral), which increases overall volume and fullness of the breasts. Placing the implant below the muscle provides the most natural look and feel and reduces the chance of hardened breasts.

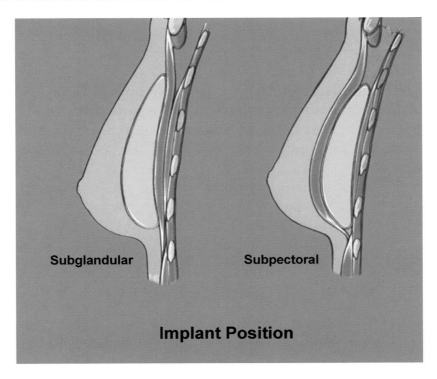

Subglandular   Subpectoral

Implant Position

Breast implant position (above vs. below the pectoralis major muscle)

All implants are manmade and have a maximum lifespan of ten to fifteen years, so they will need to be replaced during your lifetime. This needs to be discussed with your surgeon. After eight to ten years, I suggest doing a combination of a mammogram with a focused ultrasound study or a dedicated breast MRI to assess implant ruptures if you have silicone gel implants.

Have your surgeon advise you on where he or she thinks the optimal approach for the incision should be for your implants. You must fully understand the benefits and risks of having breast implants. Your implants will need to be replaced in approximately ten to fifteen years. Regular follow-up appointments are suggested with your surgeon—at least once a year. Ultimately, you are the one who has to be happy and happiness requires being informed. ***Don't obsess over the scars, as they will fade with time. Let your choice be guided by your surgeon to achieve the best balance, symmetry, and most natural appearance.***

Implant Size and Sizing

When it comes to implant sizing, you again have options—but you must work with your surgeon to consider your chest wall shape, your body form, your lifestyle, your natural foundation, and your goals. Think about how you want to ultimately look and feel with your new body.

Implants are measured by volume in terms of cc's, which refers to how much filling they contain. Unfortunately, sizing an implant is not a "trying on" process—it isn't like trying on a bra! The implant will **not** sit in a bra in the same position that it will be within the breast, where it is compressed against the body and breast tissue/pectoral muscle. You must work closely with your surgeon and let him or her direct you toward the best implant options.

In general, I advise patients not to go up more than two bra cup sizes, as anything larger can overwhelm the chest in terms of appearance, diameter, and/or width. Also, cup sizes do not equate to implant sizes—it varies from patient to patient according to the size and shape of the bust and body. Breast augmentation is indicated primarily for those who have insufficient breast volume and want superior fullness.

During consultation for breast augmentation, I discuss with my patients their goals to optimize reshaping and sizing of the breasts. If the goals are extremely out of line with what would look natural and harmonious, I do not recommend surgery. For example, I saw a twenty-two-year-old woman who weighed one hundred and ten pounds. She had almost no breast tissue and a narrow breast diameter, but she wanted a full D-cup because of her new boyfriend's urging. I took a long deep breath and explained to her that her motivations, let alone her desires, were not in line with her overall small body frame. The same woman came back to see me nine months later. She had broken up with the boyfriend and decided upon a realistic augmentation for her chest and body. Today, she is delighted with her more natural C-cup breasts and respects the beauty of her own body.

When you see your surgeon, bring in photos that inspire you—based on women with similar characteristics and qualities. This can be helpful, but realize that photos and research cannot guarantee an identical or exact outcome. My job is to make you happy in the body you already have, not discourage you with someone else's seemingly ideal form.

Implant Types: Saline vs. Silicone

In the United States, breast implants have either a saline solution or silicone gel inside. While there are a few key differences, both types of implants share many things in common. They both have a lifespan of ten to fifteen years, are FDA-approved, and are safe, though each carries a small risk of complications (as do all implants.) The often-quoted rupture or contracture rate is about 1 percent per year. Although this does mean the implant has to be removed, it is not a medical emergency. The implant can be removed and replaced in one procedure.

Silicone implants tend to be more expensive than saline implants, require larger incisions to be placed, and may require a more involved procedure—the tradeoff is that they will usually bring a more natural and realistic feel. Silicone implants are especially valuable for patients with little or no breast tissue.

Similarities in Saline and Silicone Implants:

- Both have a silicone outer shell

- Both last approximately ten to fifteen years

- Both are FDA-approved for breast augmentation

- Both have excellent safety records (as published in scientific literature)

Silicone and saline implants are both considered to be very safe. However, the FDA allows only saline implants to be used for cosmetic breast augmentation patients between the ages of eighteen and twenty-two. FDA guidelines are suggestions only, and are not based on scientific studies. In the event of rupture, the saline (salt water) will simply be absorbed into the body.

In women with ample breast tissue, the look and feel of the saline implant will be very similar to silicone implants—the combination of the muscle and the breast tissue overlaying the implant allows the implant to add volume without substantially changing the look or feel of the overlying breast tissue.

Both saline and silicone implants should be placed beneath the muscle in order to prevent rippling and hardening. If you have little breast tissue, I recommend that you opt for a smooth silicone gel round implant as they have less chance of visible rippling.

In the event of a saline implant rupture, they will deflate, resulting in an unmistakable change in the shape of the breast. Saline solution poses no health risks and is harmlessly taken in by the body.

However, silicone gel implants can rupture "silently"—without any overt warning—over time. The FDA recommends having an MRI scan beginning three years post-op and then every two years thereafter. I usually recommend another MRI after ten years with a silicone implant. That way, we can tell the status of the implant and act accordingly.

Differences in Saline and Silicone Implants:

Saline:

- Lower incidence of hardening

- Ruptures immediately detectable as saline is quickly, but harmlessly, absorbed by the body, resulting in deflation

- Inserted and replaced through a smaller incision

- May have a less natural feel in patients with little or no breast tissue

- Replacement is a simple procedure

- Slightly higher incidence of drooping, bottoming out, and lowering the breast fold

Silicone:

- Feel and look very natural

- Higher incidence of hardening

- Ruptures more difficult to detect, requiring monitoring

- Larger incision required for insertion

- Higher cost implant

- Replacement is a more involved procedure

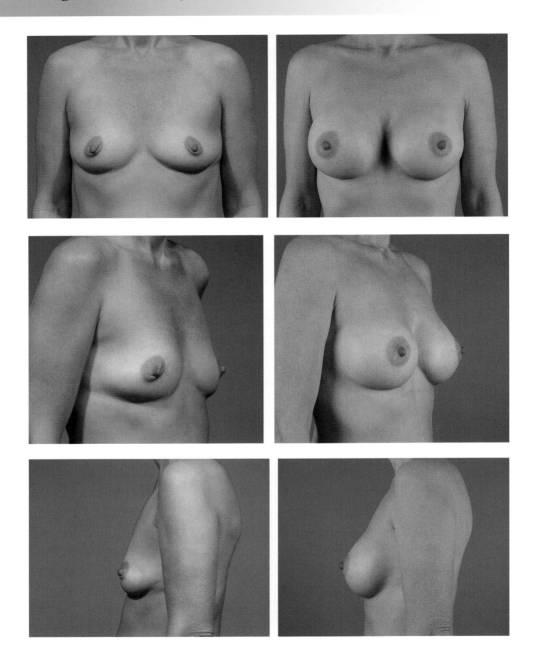

This patient had smooth silicone implants placed subpectorally via inframammary incisions – patient had inadequate breast tissue

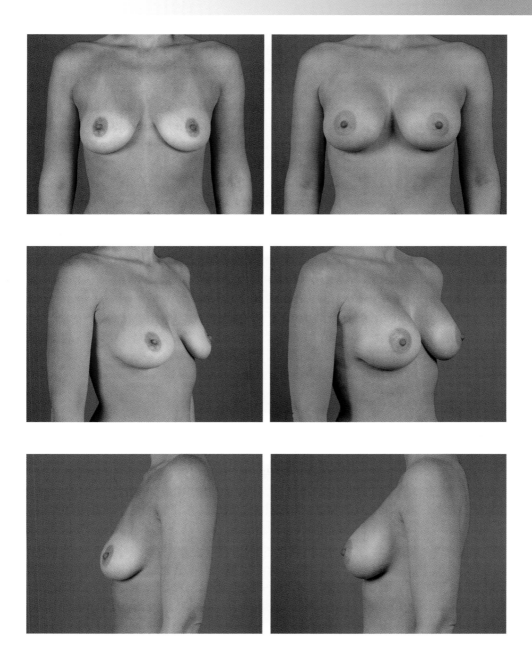

This patient had saline implants with an excellent result as she had adequate breast tissue

Implant hardening (capsular contracture) is more common with silicone implants than saline ones. Saline implants have less incidence of capsular contracture, but they also present a slightly higher incidence of drooping, bottoming out, and lowering the breast fold over time. Most of the time smooth implants are used rather than textured as they look and feel more natural. Textured implants are generally used in patients with recurrent breast hardening.

These implant differences are notable and worth consideration. Keep in mind, though, that the patient satisfaction rate is very high for both saline and silicone implants. Breast enhancement is a very common procedure. **As Dr. Rohrich states, no breast implant lasts forever, and choosing to have breast augmentation brings regular maintenance—no matter what type of implant. Both saline and silicone implants look and feel good; ask your expert plastic surgeon for guidance as to which is best for you.** *Copy the summary below and take it to your breast augmentation consult. You will find it invaluable. If the plastic surgeon you meet isn't open to this kind of discussion, go elsewhere!*

Recovery From Breast Augmentation

For the vast majority of patients, breast augmentation procedures are short and recuperation is relatively easy compared to other plastic surgery procedures. They are most often performed as outpatient procedures, and most patients go home on the very same day. Most patients will feel a slight tightness or soreness for a few days in the chest area. This is very natural. You will be instructed to wear a specialized support bra, and never an underwire bra, for three to four weeks. Most other activities can be resumed after that time. Remember to get clearance from your surgeon.

*****Contrary to popular rumor, implants do not complicate breast cancer screenings—especially with today's advanced mammogram, sonogram, and MRI techniques. Of course, you do want to let your breast imaging center know that you have implants prior to screening.***

The risks are very similar to those of other surgeries: infection, bleed-ing, scarring, and asymmetry are all possible, so you want to find a sur-geon with the highest skill and most comprehensive—and breast-spe-cific—experience. The most frequent—and most preventable—problem with breast augmentation is not getting the size you want. This can occur frequently to anyone who goes "shopping" for the doctor with the lowest price who may be inexperienced and may not even be a plastic surgeon. While a breast augmentation procedure is common, it's not a one-size-fits-all purchase.

Keep your entire body in mind when selecting an implant size. Listen to your surgeon and let him or her counsel you as to how your desires fit realistically. If you are worried about price, keep in mind that complica-tions will overwhelm any upfront costs. It's a lot cheaper to have it done right the first time! Not to mention the discomfort and upset of having to redo an imperfectly performed procedure.

I recently saw a woman who had implants done in an office setting by an internist. She developed a life-threatening infection that sent her to the emergency room in the middle of the night. We removed the implants and placed her on IV antibiotics for two weeks. She had to wait almost a full year to have her implants replaced. I performed the procedure in a proper and sterile operating room environment, unlike her previ-ous experience. She looks great now, but she was lucky. I don't want to scare you, but merely entice you to do your research and select the cor-rect board certified plastic surgeon first and foremost with expertise in breast surgery.

Risks/Capsular Contracture (Breast Implant Hardness)

In addition to the usual risks of infection, bleeding, and excessive scarring, breast implant patients have the additional risk of capsu-lar contracture. This is a condition that occurs in a small percentage of breast-implant patients, most frequently in woman who have had breast implants for a long time. The problem arises when the body is too aggressive in sealing off the implant and the collagen fibers tighten around and squeeze the implants. This can result in breasts that are too firm, misshapen, and—in severe cases—painful.

In the event of capsular contracture, your surgeon may need to re-move the implant and reshape the breast. A new implant may be insert-ed at this time. In these situations, I generally use a textured implant, because it has been shown to have less incidence of recurrent breast hardness.

One cannot prevent capsular contracture; however, one can start with massaging and moving the implant around within three to five days of the procedure. Make this a regular habit so you can keep a larg-er pocket for your implant to move around freely and naturally.

Understand that capsular contracture is largely a phenomenon de-termined by your own genetics. If your surgeon has reason to believe you are at risk for hardening, you can simply choose an implant type (a textured saline implant placed below the muscle) that further mini-mizes the chance for capsular contracture.

Breast Lift vs. Breast Lift Plus Augmentation: When and Why

Loss of breast volume usually leads to breast ptosis or drooping of the breasts. As women age, hormonal changes make drooping extremely common, though it also affects some younger women, especially after pregnancy and breastfeeding. Weight loss is also a common cause of drooping, because excess fat leads to excess skin—when the weight is lost, the skin remains, and that can lead to sagging.

A lift will correct drooping by volumetrically reshaping the breasts, which gives drooping breasts a more youthful appearance.

There is a very simple self-diagnostic test to identify a case of droop-ing breasts: the Pencil Test.

Place a pencil as high as you can inside the underneath breast fold. If the pencil stays held in the fold under your breast when you let go, then you likely have the beginning of drooping and/or volume loss in your breast. If the nipple is below the pencil, you almost certainly have substantial ptosis and may be a prime candidate for a breast lift.

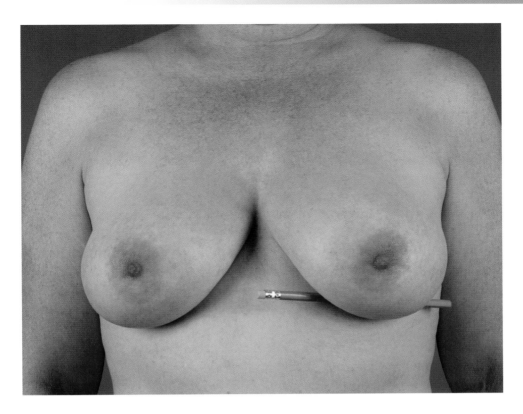

The "Pencil Test" reveals this patient may benefit from a breast lift

The three different types of breast lift incisions are as follows:

1. *Periareolor Incision:* This incision follows the outside of the areola and is usually only used in patients with larger areolas who need a very small lift. It has limited application in most patients.

2. *Vertical Breast Reduction Incision:* This incision also tracks the outside of the areola but also includes a vertical incision that runs from the nipple to the breast fold. This is used in patients with minimal to moderate ptosis only.

3. *The Inverted-T Incision:* This is like the vertical incision but also includes a horizontal incision across the breast fold, creating a T or anchor-shaped pattern. This is the most common and reliable incision with the most predictable results.

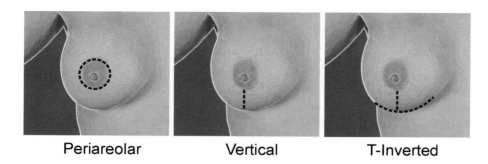

Periareolar	Vertical	T-Inverted

Commonly used breast lift incisions

Which technique is right for you? That depends on the amount of breast volume and tissue and the degree of ptosis you have. The more drooping there is to correct, the more incisions you will need in order to achieve a lift with the proper balance.

Breast enhancement (or reshaping, etc.) is like any other surgery, in that you need to be patient and let the body do its job to heal. Many patients are concerned about the scars, and you should have this frank discussion with your surgeon. The amount of scarring varies with each case and is difficult to predict. Ethnic patients may have slightly more visible and longer lasting scars due to differences in skin color and tone. Scarring is unavoidable, but the scars will mature and fade with the passage of time.

A breast lift can be performed as an isolated procedure that will remove excess skin, boost volume, reshape the breasts, and move the nipple back into a natural position. **However, a breast lift does not address the lost volume in the upper breast that contributes to breast ptosis in the first place. To achieve this, consider having breast augmentation in combination with your breast lift.**

Some patients, for whatever reason, do not want to have an implant. This is a personal choice. Of course, you can always elect for breast augmentation after your breast lift, if you should decide you want more fullness. However, it is more convenient and more expedient to do both procedures simultaneously.

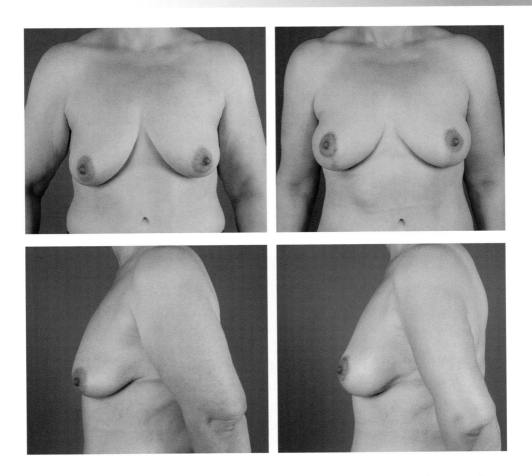

Breast augmentation and lift in a postpartum patient with smooth round 200 cc silicone gel implants

Recovery From a Breast Lift

A breast lift is often done as an outpatient procedure, but I frequently recommend an overnight stay in our nursing facility. The actual breast lift surgery takes a little longer—about two to three hours. Recovery time is similar to that of breast augmentation. You can resume your normal routine within three to four weeks. Your surgeon may put in drains during the procedure to prevent swelling and fluid accumulation—these will be removed after a day or two.

In general, I suggest my patients wait until after having their children to have a breast lift, as pregnancy and breastfeeding can change the appearance and structure of the breast.

A woman's body changes with the passage of time, including, of course, her breasts. Over time, implants and a breast lift will need to be reassessed and redone (approximately ten to fifteen years) as part of healthy personal maintenance. Care issues will be inevitable, and you want to have a long-term connection with your plastic surgeon so he or she can evaluate your specific needs and talk to you about what is to be expected over time.

Breast Lifts—What Are the Risks?

Some risks with lifts are similar to augmentation—excess swelling, bleeding, scarring, and breast asymmetry—if not performed properly. As always, choosing a high quality surgeon you trust minimizes these risks. **An augmentation/mastopexy (augment/breast lift done together) is a more complicated operation than augmentation alone, so there is a higher risk for some complications, particularly loss of nipple sensation and scarring.** Therefore, you should not "over-augment" when doing a lift, as it may increase the chance of skin loss. If you smoke, you should not have this procedure as the risks of complications are too high. You need to stop smoking for four weeks prior to surgery so that you maximize your healing post-op. The key is to emphasize balance and breast/body proportion.

Breast Reduction

Breast reduction candidates are some of my happiest patients—they report higher satisfaction than just about any other class of patient. For anyone suffering from macromastia or excessive breast size, this will come as no surprise. There are significant physical and psychological components to excessive breast size. They experience symptoms such as shoulder, neck, and back pain, as well as bra-strap ribbing, painful grooves in the shoulder, and skin irritation. The psychological symptoms are not to be ignored, either; patients often come to me with feelings of embarrassment, unattractiveness, and deep self-consciousness.

Fortunately, a breast reduction can eliminate many of these symptoms, both physical and psychological, by making the breasts smaller, lighter, and more in balance with a person's body type. Neck, back, and shoulder pain are usually alleviated once the stress of the extra weight is reduced. There is no reason to suffer with macromastia, and doing so can be detrimental to your long-term health.

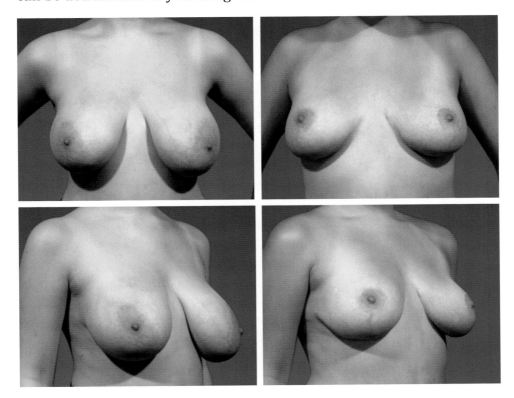

This patient had breast reduction using inverted-T incision for greatly improved breast shape and contour as well as an improved body image

Here are the techniques used in breast reduction surgery:

- **The Inverted-T Incision:** This is the traditional and most common incision. It involves making an opening around and below the areola, along the breast fold (making an upside-down "T" below the nipple). This technique is particularly well suited to patients who are removing a large volume of breast tissue as it allows for the skin to be tightened evenly—and attractively—even after a substantial amount of tissue has been excised. (It is similar to the incision for a breast lift.)

- **Vertical Breast Reduction Incision:** This method has been gaining in popularity during recent years. This incision also goes around and down from the areola, but does not go across the breast fold. It has several distinct advantages, most obviously that there is no scar on the underside of the breast. Also, it provides a slightly rounder, more natural and youthful-looking breast than the inverted-T incision in some patients—namely, those patients having small to moderate breast reductions. The catch is that the technique is not suitable for those having large-size reductions— the inverted-T is still the gold standard.

- **Liposuction**

    a. *Breast Liposuction (Female):* This practice uses liposuction only to remove fat from the breast. This is by far the least invasive, but cannot remove the excess skin. It, therefore, has limited use in reducing breast size. This procedure is generally used for patients who want to remove a small amount of fat. It is best for younger women who have soft breasts and good skin tone, so the skin cooperates and tightens on its own during the post-op period.

    b. *Liposuction Breast Reduction (Male):* Liposuction is the primary and preferred treatment in the management of male breast enlargement, which is called **gynecomastia**. (See Chapter 2 for example.) This is the most common male breast problem, seen in up to 20 percent of males, beginning at puberty. Most of the time the cause is unknown and benign.

Breast reduction is not only an aesthetic surgery, but also a corrective medical procedure that is often covered by insurance. Speak with both your surgeon and your insurance company to see what help may be provided—often, it is merely a matter of having the procedure defined in medical terms.

As with breast augmentation and lifting, breast reduction can be an outpatient procedure performed under general anesthesia. You will be able to go home on the same day and can get back to regular exercise and activity in three to four weeks. A supportive bra is recommended for at least the first four weeks.

The risks are similar to those experienced with a breast lift, as similar incisions are made. So, we again remind you to choose carefully when selecting your plastic surgeon.

Breast reduction, breast lifts, and breast augmentation are methods of correcting similar problems—breasts that are out of proportion with the body. The difference is in the type of patient—one will be a woman who feels her breasts are too large for her frame, caused by excessive breast tissue (breast overgrowth), while another feels her breasts droop too much (breast ptosis). The augmentation woman wants to add volume, as she lacks sufficient tissue. The outcome and goals for all these operations are relatively similar: well-proportioned, natural-looking breasts with ample—but not excessive—volume.

Breast Reconstruction Options– From Cosmetic to Reconstruction

One in eight American women is diagnosed with breast cancer. The treatment of breast cancer has moved toward breast-conserving therapy, but one-third of breast cancer patients still require mastectomies. Reconstructive breast surgery is, therefore, an integral part of cancer treatment. It is a significant part of physical and emotional healing for women who have undergone mastectomies. Breast reconstruction following cancer and mastectomy is very similar to the purely cosmetic augmentation and reshaping surgeries. The desired surgical outcome is the same across all of these procedures: giving the patient the best, most natural-appearing breasts possible. The goal is to help cancer survivors with mastectomies complete the healing process by restoring an emotional sense of wholeness, and physical sense of feeling complete.

If you are considering breast reconstruction, it is important to understand the benefits and limitations. We are fortunate today to have many great reconstructive options available. With the guidance of a good surgeon well versed in breast reconstruction, you will be able to select the options that are best suited to your specific body and needs.

There are three main types of breast reconstruction procedures:

- *Implant-Based Reconstruction:* This type of breast reconstruction involves the restoration of the breast using a breast implant. The procedure may be delayed or done immediately.

- *Combination of Implant and Autologous Tissue Reconstruction:* This combination option utilizes both an implant and tissue taken from the back to reconstruct the breast.

- *Autologous Tissue Breast Reconstruction:* These procedures use your body's own fat instead of a breast implant in order to reconstruct and fill the breast. The donor tissue may be taken from your abdomen, buttock, or thighs and consists of only fat and skin—there is no need to sacrifice important muscle tissue from elsewhere in the body. These procedures have been refined in recent times to provide a much more natural result than they once did.

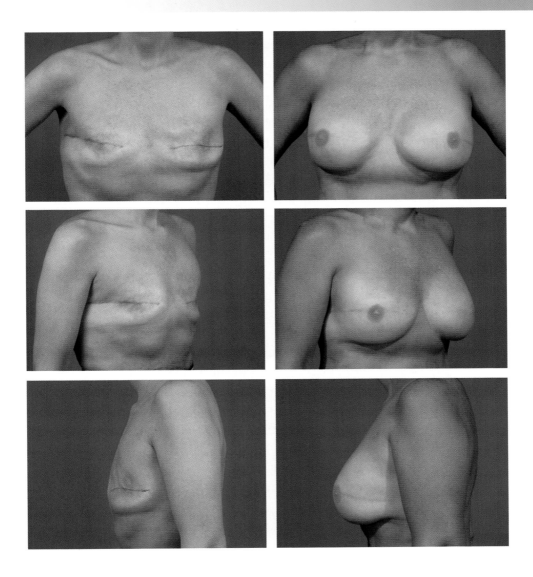

Bilateral mastectomy patient who underwent breast reconstruction using textured silicone gel implants and nipple reconstruction with areolar tattooing

Five Key Points to Remember:

1. Breast enhancement is done to create a more balanced and natural-looking breast through augmentation (when there is too little tissue), reduction (when there is too much breast tissue), and breast lifting (to correct too much breast drooping). Augmentation and reduction are done in combination with a breast lift when there is both drooping and too little or too much breast volume, respectively.

2. There is no one perfect size or shape of breast—your plastic surgeon will act as a guide to help identify a size and shape appropriate to your body.

3. Make sure you discuss the following four topics with your plastic surgeon so you understand your options:
   a. Types of incisions (inframammary/transaxillary/periareolar)
   b. Implant types (saline/silicone and textured/smooth surface)
   c. Implant size/sizing
   d. Risks (such as hardening/capsular contracture)

4. Breast reconstruction, surgical reconstruction of the breast after mastectomy, shares the same goals as other cosmetic breast procedures: to restore the breasts to a natural and balanced appearance in order to improve the patient's physical and emotional well-being.

5. For all of these procedures, you need a plastic surgeon who is an expert in surgery of the breast and has expertise in your particular procedure.

Liposuction and Body Contouring

9

Liposuction, along with breast enhancement, is one of the most frequently performed procedures in the field of plastic surgery. Likewise, it is also one of the most misunderstood. **Contrary to popular misconception, liposuction works to reshape and contour the body in diet and exercise-resistant areas—it is not meant to shed large quantities of weight and it will not magically make you thinner.**

*Obesity is a pervasive problem in modern America and a huge healthcare issue that affects us in both physical and emotional ways. **Losing weight is no easy task; the diets, ideas, and disciplines touted by the media are mostly just empty marketing. So what can you do? In this chapter, we want to help you navigate the lifelong changes you need, especially when considering liposuction or body contouring.***

Do the three question Mirror Test again, this time with your whole body in mind. First, give yourself a compliment. But perhaps you've let yourself go a little and have not been the best steward of your body. You may not love what you see in the mirror, but know you can do something to change that. No matter where you are in life, regardless of the frustration you may feel, there are solutions and this can be your time. Each day is a new opportunity to take control of how you look and feel.

You and your expert body contouring plastic surgeon will work together to improve the look of your body and restore it to its natural and beautiful shape. Sometimes, though, liposuction isn't the answer. A woman came to my office recently for liposuction. She weighed 160 pounds and told me that she wanted to "get thin." She said the fad diets hadn't worked—nothing had helped. She had not tried the basics of healthy nutrition and regular exercise. She was not a candidate for liposuction or body contouring because hers was a problem of basic lifestyle.

Unfortunately, there are no procedures that will provide a shortcut here. The only answer is good nutrition (not another fad diet) and exercise that will pave the way for lifelong good health. Short-term diets don't work, unless you change your lifestyle (see Lifelong Cycle of Body Beauty), because you simply put the pounds back on when you go back to your old ways. The surgeon can only put in half of the work through liposuction—you, the patient, must contribute the other half through lifestyle and diet changes.

I did a survey of my body-contouring patients on the success of their individual liposuctions. The findings confirmed that permanent changes in lifestyle (diet and exercise) significantly improved surgical results. Among patients who adjusted their lifestyles, there was a 90 percent real success rate over the long term. However, those who made no other changes reported only a 60 percent success rate. There's simply no use in making an investment in yourself if you are not willing to follow through long-term.

Dr. Rohrich makes a critical point here if you are considering liposuction. **If you want real results, focus on inches, not pounds! Liposuction will reshape your body, but you have to lose the pounds first. The purpose of liposuction is to combine this body-contouring procedure with great nutrition, which will refine and boost your change in lifestyle.**

An acquaintance of mine was nearly sixty pounds heavier than she needed to be. She saw a surgeon who did not require her to lose any weight before the procedure. She felt that liposuction would be her "ticket to weight loss" and that everything would be just fine. But it's now two years later and she still has not lost the weight, nor made any changes to her overall nutritional diet and lifestyle. These two things go hand in hand. Getting liposuction without adopting a healthier, better lifestyle and diet is pointless. Your newly sculpted figure will simply disappear under fat tissue if you gain substantial weight back after the surgery. It is normal to have 5 to 10 percent fluctuations in weight, especially due to pregnancy

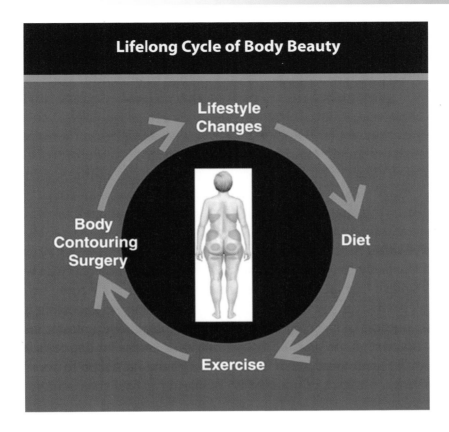

and aging (both of which cause hormonal changes), but any more than this is detrimental and can reduce the major gains made through surgery.

If you bought a luxury car, you'd treat it very well. You would schedule regular maintenance to make sure it keeps running well. Yet people often don't take the same care with their bodies and their surgical results, but the principle is the same. It's your BODY, after all—take care of it and it will make you happier than almost anything.

For detailed information on staying healthy and maintaining your results, see Chapter 13.

What Liposuction Can Do for You— If You Find the Right Surgeon

You should make every effort to lose your excess weight before surgery. This is referred to as the Lifelong Cycle of Body Beauty. **The ideal**

candidate will be within 10 to 15 percent of their ideal body weight before undergoing any type of body-contouring procedures or liposuction. Ideally, you want to be able to maintain this weight loss for a substantial time—up to a year is best—before having liposuction.

This procedure is ideal for patients who are physically active and maintain a proper diet and for those who are close to their ideal weight, but cannot manage to get rid of the extra paunch, saddlebags, excess flab, or other such excess fat in the body. Many patients come in with complaints for the most common exercise-resistant areas—the love handles and inner and outer thighs.

Weight loss through proper diet and exercise isn't always enough to return the body to its natural and youthful shape, especially as we age. This is where liposuction and body-contouring surgery come into play, and this is why we say that these procedures focus on shedding inches, not just pounds of fat. Your skilled and carefully chosen plastic surgeon will literally reshape your body by removing excess fat deposits and fat cells. At the same time, he or she will sculpt the fat tissue to accentuate the natural contours of your body, restoring it to a trim and youthful appearance.

Liposuction is not an easy procedure. It saddens me to see amateurs or so-called, self-designated cosmetic surgeons operate and literally experiment with body contouring on unsuspecting patients. **They rely on unproven technology rather than skill and training to potentially obtain results.** Technology is our artistic tool, but the tool matters less than the "artist"—the body contouring plastic surgeon's expertise is what counts. True talent and expertise require years of practice and training to develop. Find a true expert body contouring plastic surgeon. As always, remember to ask the ***Three Magic Questions*** (see Chapter 3).

Am I a Candidate for Liposuction Alone?

This is a key question, and the easy way to determine the answer is again the Mirror Test. If you can grasp your fat between your hands—if you have too much skin—you are not a candidate. For example, you may need a tummy tuck if you can do this grasp test on your tummy or abdominal wall area.

There is no such thing as a simple "spot" liposuction, as fat deposits are not isolated within the body. The key to obtaining a well-sculpted figure is for the plastic surgeon to consider the body as a whole. As a body-contouring plastic surgeon who understands the importance of restoring one's aesthetic body silhouette, I consider the whole body in a comprehensive contouring deliberation. Your body is an absolute work of art, so you need a true artist of a surgeon to restore it.

Not long ago, a prospective patient told me she "just wanted liposuction on her outer thighs only." However, she also had a problem with excess fat layered on her trunk and belly, as well as in the thighs. If I only worked on her thighs, it would have left her with a strange body shape and masculinized body form. She could not foresee the need for more comprehensive work, as the thighs were the one area she was focused on fixing. I imaged the procedure she wanted and she quickly saw that she needed more than spot liposuction to resolve all issues to prevent her having a masculinized figure change. I performed a complete body sculpting on her so she retained and enhanced her female body silhouette. The real lesson here is to not fix one problem only—for example, only doing spot liposuction, and thereby creating another larger problem (masculinizing the female silhouette).

Liposuction alone will not remove cellulite and it can even make it worse, especially if your surgeon overdoes the liposuction. If you have significant cellulite or dimpling, especially in the buttocks, a surgeon can refill this as needed with fat reinjections for *reshaping.* A liposuction procedure can be an ideal time to do this, as fat removed from one area can be transferred to another to refill lost volume and smooth out the appearance of cellulite.

Types of Liposuction Procedures—What Are Your Options?

Liposuction is performed by making multiple small incisions to treat specific fat deposits across the entire body. At each incision, your surgeon will insert a cannula, a tube for breaking up and removing excess fat cells.

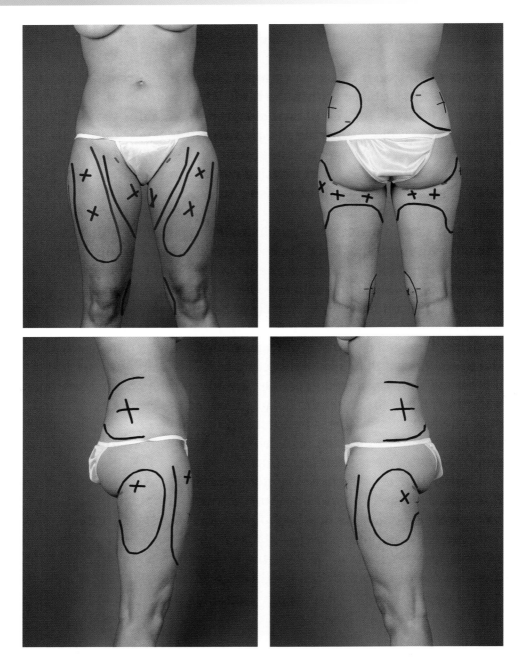

Typical markings for three-dimensional (3-D) lower body liposuction

Fat cells play an important role in metabolism as storage and energy depots, but when you gain too much weight, they swell and distort your figure. **Here is a scientific fact: You are born with a set number of fat cells that remain largely unchanged after puberty. As you age and gain weight, you do not gain more cells, but the cells you do have** *expand*. **When you lose weight, the cells contract and become smaller, but the total number remains the same.** When you are near your ideal body weight, liposuction will remove many of these fat cells permanently. This is why you really want to be in the best shape possible before having liposuction (or any type of body-contouring surgery). Weight gain or weight loss causes expansion and contraction of your body, and this will negatively alter the appearance of the fine-finessed sculpting performed by your surgeon.

There are several liposuction methods and techniques. The traditional method is **suction-assisted liposuction**, which uses a cannula inserted under the skin through small incisions to literally vacuum excess fat cells from the body.

The key to a natural appearance in performing liposuction is *less is more*. I do not over-correct—I remove only the precise amount of fat necessary to re-sculpt the body. Overcorrection causes deformities that are hard to correct.

The newer techniques are simply variations of a regular suction-assisted technique. For example, some surgeons use **power-assisted liposuction** in which the cannula is automated to move back and forth. This reduces the amount of manual movements the surgeon must make and can make it faster and easier to remove fat and sculpt the body.

Another excellent liposuction method is **ultrasound-assisted liposuction** (UAL), which uses ultrasound shockwaves to melt and liquefy the fat in place, making it easier to suction via the cannula. This is especially effective if the targeted fat deposit is comprised of thick and fibrous tissue such as in the back and breasts. This type of liposuction can also be used in secondary contouring for previous liposuction patients. Men benefit from ultrasound-assisted liposuction as they are much harder to work on because their fat is more fibrous.

One of the most highly marketed types of liposuction is **laser liposuction**, although there is no definitive data available on success rates.

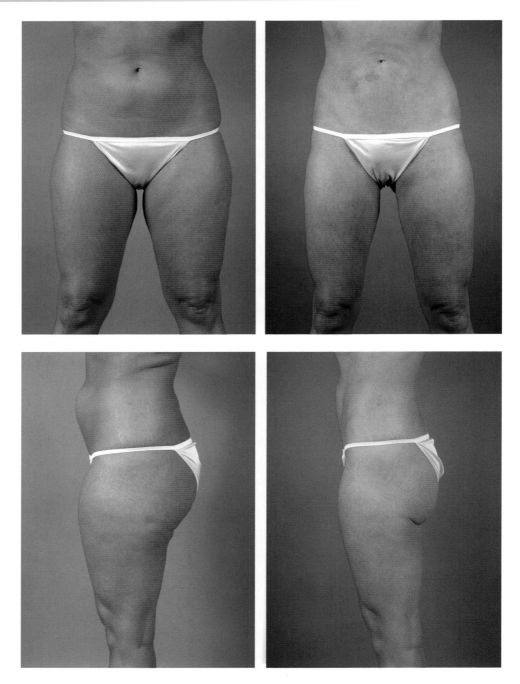

Patient underwent 3-D liposuction of thighs and flanks with sustained post-op diet/exercise

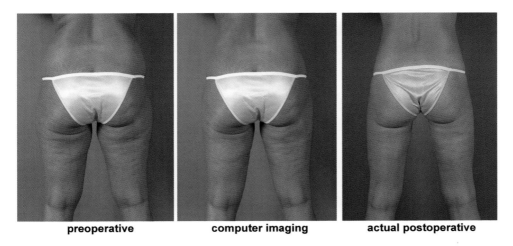

| preoperative | computer imaging | actual postoperative |

Computer imaging to show possible post-op results as well as actual post-op results with thigh and flank liposuction

These are before-and-after photos of an ideal candidate who saw good results. Always ask to see such photos of patients so you have a visual reference for how well the doctor performs.

Make sure you discuss with your plastic surgeon the areas of the body that are most effectively treated with liposuction and safe to work on. These include the abdomen, buttocks, inner and outer thighs, flanks, hips, and upper arms. I use circumferential body contouring, also known as 3-D contouring, and carefully and conservatively suction all the way around the thigh to restore the cosmetic shape.

Safety and Risks—What You Need to Know

A single session of liposuction rarely lasts more than three hours. The key to a successful surgery is to maximize safety and efficiency so the surgeon can remove as much fat as possible in the scheduled time frame. Have a candid conversation with your surgeon about the techniques and methods that are suitable for you.

General anesthesia is, in my opinion, vitally important to achieve outcomes safely in contouring procedures. If you prefer *not* to be put under general anesthesia, talk with your surgeon and anesthesiologist about other options. Most plastic surgeons prefer to use general anesthesia for optimal patient comfort and patient safety.

Recovery From Liposuction

Liposuction of less than six pounds of fat removal is usually performed on an outpatient basis. If a greater amount needs to be removed, I highly recommend staying in an aftercare facility with 24/7 nursing care. (You only lose about 50 percent of the weight from the amount of fat removed.) We make sure to get the patient up and walking almost immediately after the surgery, as it helps with circulation and healing and prevents post-op complications.

After the operation, you will be fitted with a specialized protective garment that fits your body snugly (see below).

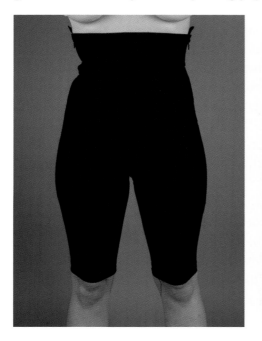 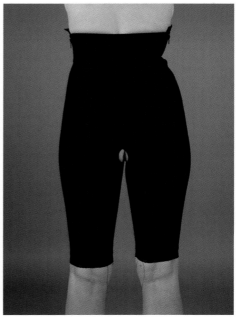

Post-operative compression garments

These garments help minimize bruising and swelling and allow for optimal wound healing. My patients wear a compression garment after surgery, which is removed in my office on day three. Patients then wear compression garments day and night for two weeks and then for another two weeks only at night. At this point, the garment can be discontinued, though many patients continue wearing them for up to a few months post-op for comfort.

Your incisions and all of the liposuctioned areas will be firm and numb up to two or three months after surgery. You can resume most activities—including exercise—in three to four weeks, but always consult with your surgeon first. Your liposuction areas will also feel numb and tingle for six to twelve weeks. This is normal. You need to get your body moving as quickly as possible because staying active helps your new contours settle.

Maintaining a healthy weight is essential for real results; failure to take care of yourself will negate the surgery completely. Stay motivated and stay vigilant—liposuction is only one small part of the process. You want to maintain a normal body weight to keep your results. **Please do not weigh yourself for at least three weeks as you may have early weight gain from post-op surgical swelling. This is normal!**

Tummy Tucks—What Are They For? When Do You Need One?

An abdominoplasty, or a tummy tuck, is a common body-contouring procedure that removes excess loose skin in the abdominal area. Skin expands, loses tone, and sags as we age, fluctuate in weight, or bear children. The abdominal area is especially susceptible to expansion and sagging in those who tend to carry weight in their belly. Abdominoplasty is often coupled with some love handle or flank liposuction for true mid-trunk shaping as part of a comprehensive body-contouring plan. Successful abdominoplasty removes excess skin, sculpts underlying fat, and in some cases, involves the tightening of the underlying muscles.

Am I a Candidate?

You should also be within 10 to 15 percent of your ideal body weight before having a tummy tuck. The best way to tell if you need a tummy tuck is simply to glance in the mirror and take this three question Mirror Test:

1. Is the skin loose and sagging?

2. Can you grasp skin above and below your belly button?

3. Do you have extra skin folds above your belly button when you sit down?

If the answer to all of these questions is no, you may only need liposuction and not tightening of the skin. However, if you do have extra skin, you are a candidate for a tummy tuck. The positive Grasp Test is an easy and effective diagnostic tool.

If you have recently lost weight or have had children, consider trying to maintain your current weight for a year before having the procedure, because gaining weight will compromise your results. This is true of all body-contouring procedures. For the same reason, you should have a tummy tuck done only after having all of your children, as pregnancy causes hormonal changes which can affect weight—not to mention the new baby stretching the abdominal area.

Overall health is just as important as your weight. **If you are a smoker, have significant scarring in your abdomen, or have a significant medical condition, you are not a candidate for this procedure. Smokers have a high risk of complications. I require patients to quit smoking for at least four to six weeks before their surgery.**

The recovery time for a tummy tuck is normally two to three weeks. I have all my patients out of bed and moving immediately after surgery and often (up to eight times per day) and have them walking within three to five days. Lying in bed too long increases your risk for blood clots.

A new and very useful recent advancement in patient care is **Exparel®**, a local anesthetic with excellent, long-lasting results. It has

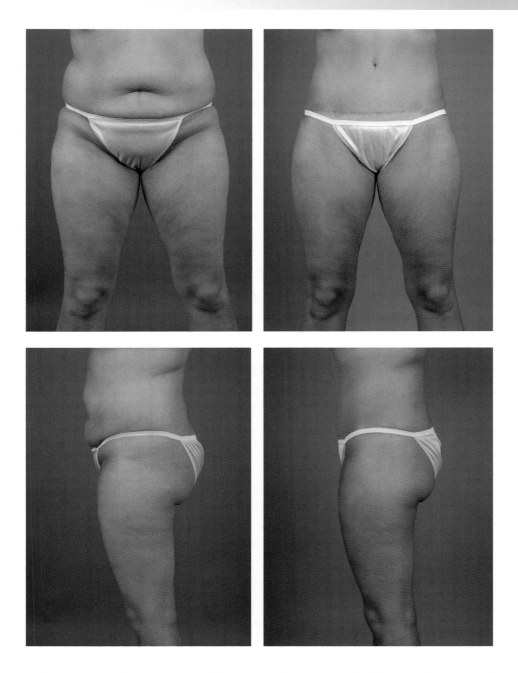

A tummy tuck patient with improved contour of abdominal area and flanks. Note how the patient has restored shape to the trunk and thigh areas.

remarkable benefits in the recovery period by reducing pain in the first few post-op days.

Liposuction, like weight loss, may make sagging skin worse! One of my friends had liposuction after having three children, but what she needed was a tummy tuck. After the liposuction, the skin was actually looser because she had less fat volume underneath. Thankfully, Dr. Rohrich then did her tummy tuck and flank liposuction to reshape her, and she now looks and feels better than ever. Do not make this same mistake—get the right procedure. Remember, this requires knowledge and research and a surgeon who focuses on your whole body.

There are several different classes of abdominoplasty procedures that are indicated for different degrees of excess skin. These are the two most common procedures:

- *Mini-Abdominoplasty:* Patients who only have extra skin and fat below, but not above the navel are ideal candidates for a mini-abdominoplasty. This kind of work targets only sagging skin below the navel. Only a small subset of abdominoplasty patients should have this procedure done; usually those who have not had children and thus do not have any diastasis (when the abdominal muscles spread) from pregnancy. Instead, the extra skin below the navel is due to weight gain or weight loss. **Incision scars are similar to those of a full abdominoplasty, but are usually shorter and limited to the area below the belly button only where the skin is removed.**

- *Full Abdominoplasty:* This is the traditional tummy tuck, targeting the entire abdominal area. This is for patients who have excess skin both above and below the belly button and have abdominal muscle widening from having children. Your surgeon will be able to tighten the underlying muscles in order to reverse diastasis. **The procedure requires an incision across the lower abdomen above the pubic area that generally goes from hip to hip along your bikini line. Depending on the amount of skin removed, a new location is made for the navel to keep the belly button looking natural in shape and placement. Most but not**

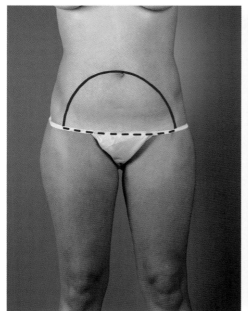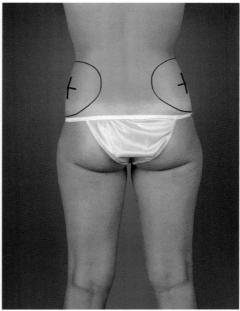

Pre-op patient markings of areas (back and flank) to be liposuctioned with a tummy tuck. Incisions are hidden in the bikini line.

all of the stretch marks below the navel can be removed during this procedure.

So, which procedure is right for you? Again, consult the mirror and do the Grasp Test. If you can pinch extra skin above and below your belly button, you're not a candidate for a mini-tuck—you may need a full traditional tummy tuck. If you can only grab excess skin below the belly button, a mini-tummy tuck may be enough to do the job.

Keep in mind that if you have had children and pregnancy has widened your stomach girth, a mini-tummy tuck probably isn't the answer. You may need at least a full tummy tuck to remove the excess skin and tighten the muscles around the abdominals that have spread.

The Mommy Makeover—What Is It and Is It Safe?

This is a marketing term for a combination tummy tuck and liposuction with breast enhancement. The name comes from its popularity

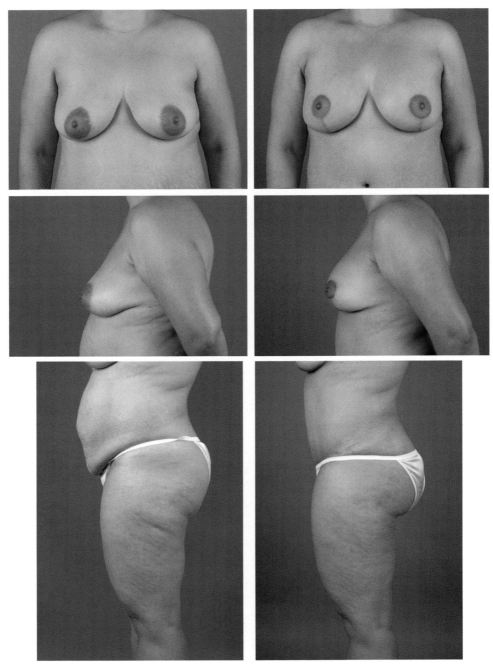

"Mommy Makeover" patient who had a breast augmentation and lift with a tummy tuck and flank liposuction. Combination procedures like these should be performed on younger, healthy patients with recovery in a high quality post-operative nursing facility.

with post-pregnancy women looking to reverse the physical changes brought on with childbearing. The name is perhaps a little silly, but definitely apt as the combination is quite effective in restoring the body to a pre-pregnancy appearance.

Combining procedures has obvious advantages—you can get everything done at once and overlap recovery times in order to minimize time away from your daily routines. However, this convenience must be carefully weighed against any effect on safety and outcome caused by a longer procedure. If the procedures will take longer than five to six hours, they need to be done in stages. I will not compromise when it comes to safety and outcome. That said, combination procedures like the Mommy Makeover can be a good choice, especially when they allow a surgeon to balance changes made in different areas of the body at the same time—this can help you achieve the greatest level of overall harmony between features.

What If I Have Experienced Significant Weight Loss?

First of all, congratulations! A significant sub-group of patients who see me for liposuction and body contouring are those who have undergone massive weight loss, which is usually defined as fifty pounds or more, often by gastric sleeves or bypass or (ideally) through exercise, diet, and portion control. Many patients complain that their bodies do not "bounce back" after shedding the weight. In particular, large amounts of excess skin result in substantial sagging, which can give the appearance of flabbiness even after the underlying fat tissue is gone.

Patients who have large amounts of excess skin due to weight loss often need a comprehensive surgical regimen and generally require total all-over body lifts. Your surgeon will make the same hip-to-hip incisions as for a tummy tuck, but they will also extend incisions into other areas of the body where the skin needs to be tightened. Normally, this requires going up the torso and may also include incisions on the backside of the arms (for an arm lift) or down the thighs and buttocks (for a thigh lift).

Medial Arm lift

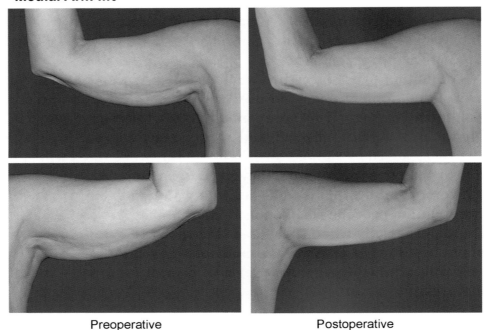

Preoperative   Postoperative

The "hidden inner arm lift"

The number, length, and placement of incisions depend on the amount of excess skin. Longer incisions from body contouring can be hidden under clothing and in the natural curves of the body. Scars are simply part of this surgical process and will mature and fade some over time. The tradeoff of having these marks is generally worth the dramatic reduction in sagging and loose skin.

This intricate and involved surgery involves the body as a whole and must usually be staged over two or three sessions, because it is generally safer to do elective surgery in less than six hours. The risk of blood clot formation and other post-op problems increases when surgery is prolonged past that time. This is especially true if you have very loose skin, as this results in a higher revision rate if further tightening and tweaking are necessary.

Every contouring surgery must be personally designed, especially if it follows a massive weight loss. Your surgeon will work with you to develop a plan to carry out your surgery over many sessions—usually two or three, but occasionally more. There are common surgical risks (clotting, bruising, bleeding, etc.), but it is generally safe as long as you are

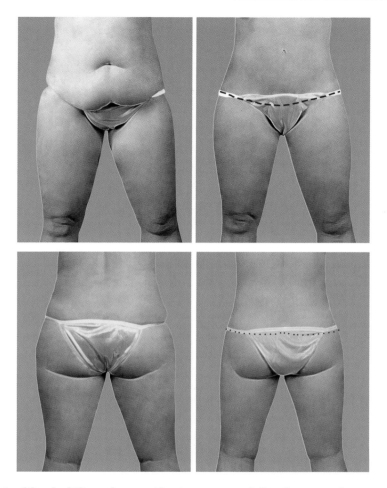

A central body lift reshapes the tummy and flank area after massive weight loss

healthy, have no significant medical history like diabetes or untreated hypertension, and you are a nonsmoker. Each session requires a three to four week recovery time. I usually space each session by about three to six months to allow the body and patient to recover fully between stages for optimal patient safety and wound healing to occur.

Massive weight loss patients must pay particular attention to their commitment to weight loss. **I recommend that massive weight loss patients do the surgery only after at least a year or two of maintained weight loss. If you regain the pounds, your skin will again stretch, completely reversing all of your surgical efforts.**

Five Key Points to Remember:

1. If you are overweight, you need to make an overall life-style change in your nutritional habits and exercise routine. Do not do any fad diets (they don't work long term). (See Chapter 13.)

2. When considering liposuction, remember the benefits are in inches, not pounds. Body contouring is not an appropriate method for weight loss and does not remove cellulite. Only diet and exercise provide the foundation for these lasting changes. Then go find your true body contouring plastic expert, and always ask the **Three Magic Questions.**

3. Body contouring, such as abdominoplasty, targets excess sagging skin above and below the belly button. Take the Grasp Test to know if you have excess loose skin. Liposuction doesn't work if you have sagging skin.

4. If you have lost an excessive amount of weight (over fifty pounds), you will likely need significant body sculpting and liposuction. Long incisions are the trade-off for improved body shape and contours. These are usually done in phases for your safety and recovery.

5. Simultaneously performing procedures is safe. Your whole procedure should last six hours or less—otherwise they must be staged. Make sure you discuss all of your surgery goals with your doctor to understand the risks and your options pre-op.

When You've Already Had Plastic Surgery:
Enhancing What Worked; Fixing What Didn't

10

Frequently throughout the book, I've made mention of helping patients dissatisfied with previous plastic surgery. In this chapter, I'd like to explore with you the options you have if you are in this all-too-common situation that I see in my daily practice. The concepts you'll find in this chapter are also intended for those whose work went well the first time, but now may need updating, or if you had a problem with an initial surgery. So if you are contemplating additional work in the same area, this chapter is meant for you.

The term for repairing prior plastic surgery is *secondary surgery*. Most secondary surgery patients fit into three categories. First, there are those who had a good experience, but need updating due to the passage of time. This generally includes patients who have had a previous well-done facelift, eye work, or a breast augmentation or lift. They come for a refresher or update after ten or so years have passed—a very normal occurrence. This is standard ongoing maintenance and care.

The **second** category is when patients had a complication from the initial surgery even when done by an expert in the field or a board certified plastic surgeon. The **third** category comprises the increasing number of patients who have undergone less-than-adequate cosmetic surgery. As the popularity of plastic surgery has increased, so has the number of so-called cosmetic doctors. As we've discussed, all too often, patients today are selecting surgeons or non-surgeons without doing the research on their background and prior work, and focusing only on marketing hype or bargain basement pricing. Alarmingly, some of these practitioners are not even real surgeons, but perform so-called "aesthetic" procedures in accordance with their own makeshift standards. You can imagine the risks of working with this kind of "professional." If this book does nothing else for you, I hope that you will stay away from these types of practitioners.

One of my revision patients had a "facelift" done by a dentist. He claimed to be trained in plastic surgery of the jaw and facial area. As you can imagine, her outcome was disastrous, giving her permanent facial nerve paralysis and terrible skin damage. I had to wait for a year to allow the area to heal before I could even attempt to fix her issues. This was a heartbreaking example of what happens when you do not get the right care. **Real plastic surgery requires a skilled, specialized expert who understands the science of the face and body and the psychology of the patient as well as how to manage complications. Remember to ask the *Three Magic Questions* and, as we discussed earlier, don't be swayed by that fancy office or those nice-looking (and all too often meaningless or misleading) certificates on the wall. As always, do your homework!**

Secondary surgeries require the doctor to blend his or her own style with the patient's previous work. It is understandably much harder to rework a previous surgery than to start fresh. If you are a candidate for such work, choose an expert surgeon who specializes in revision procedures. For example, if your rhinoplasty did not go well, you need to find a secondary rhinoplasty expert to do your next operative procedure so you can get it right this time with the highest probability for success.

New patients come to my office almost daily with a wide array of complications, ranging from subpar outcomes to significant disfigurement. I have a deep sympathy and empathy for these patients, and I work closely to resolve the damage as best as possible. Of course, by the time they see me, a patient may already have had his or her appearance altered significantly and often not in a good way. We discuss the situation and openly agree on a realistic best-case scenario. **Getting good results with secondary work can be very challenging. I reach an understanding of what can and cannot be done before I embark on operating on these patients. We all have to be on the same page!**

Some problems cannot be entirely reversed, but often most can be improved so the patient can have a more natural appearance. Patients with impaired function as well as a cosmetic deformity, such as rhinoplasty patients who have trouble breathing normally after a rhinoplasty, also have a high likelihood of finding some relief.

Understandably, patients must be reasonable about their expectations. I always discuss the real statistics with revision patients, as they have the right to know and need to be prepared. Those with significant cosmetic deformities need to have a full understanding of what can—and cannot—be done to restore shape, contour, function, and overall appearance.

As with all complex surgeries, there is a limit as to how much can be accomplished at once, especially if you are revising multiple areas. Before having the preoperative consultation (whether it be for your face, nose, breasts, or body), take a good look at yourself in the mirror. Write down the top three things you want to change or improve and share these with your revision plastic surgeon. Be very specific. Don't write something like "I want a perfect nose." We all want a perfect nose … and yet there is no such thing as a "perfect nose" or a "perfect face." My goal is to give you a more natural version of you, if possible.

I frequently turn down secondary surgery patients with unrealistic expectations. **I operate with a scalpel, not a magic wand! Revision surgery is difficult and often imperfect, and even the best surgeon may not be able to rectify one problem without creating another.** Overly ambitious and unrealistic secondary surgeons have the potential to do just that.

Do yourself a huge favor—pick the right surgeon, the first time. It may sound repetitive, but this is key! Many of my friends have asked my opinion on doctors to see for revising or fixing the work done on their nose, their face, or their breasts. It amazes me when they talk about their previous surgeons, saying they chose solely by price or the attractiveness of their websites, etc. A lot of them knew little or nothing about the individual, his or her practice, or type of specialization. There are those who spend more time shopping for a pair of shoes than for their plastic surgeon! This is your face and body—so do your research and take the time.

A person already suffering from bad plastic surgery can follow the guidelines in this chapter to be able to navigate their way toward correction of the problem. Your responsibility is to choose wisely this second time! When looking for the right surgeon for a secondary plastic surgery, consider making your search national, or even international, if that is an option for you. Secondary surgeries are demanding, and the number of surgeons who are true experts in secondary procedures such as rhinoplasty, facial rejuvenation, and body-contouring surgery is limited. So don't limit your search to surgeons only in your area—look anywhere and everywhere! Your results are forever and the price of a plane ticket will be a small investment in the larger picture for your overall happiness with your results. Remember to ask the **Three Magic Questions** *to eliminate a majority of the surgeons who are not real experts.*

Now Dr. Rohrich and I will walk you through the most common secondary procedures.

Secondary Rhinoplasty—Improving Your Nose

Secondary rhinoplasty procedures are by far the most demanding form of corrective surgeries and the most challenging plastic surgery procedure. As was discussed in Chapter 7, rhinoplasty requires precision measurable down to the millimeter. Moreover, the nose is the central focus to the balance of a person's face and is a visual anchor for all of the other features.

While primary rhinoplasty is so notably exacting, secondary procedures are even more so, but now the anatomy is scarred and may be deformed or absent! This is especially true in patients with substantial cartilage depletion. Cartilage is the connective tissue in the nose and allows for structure and support. Depleted cartilage places limits on the results a patient can realistically hope for because it gives the surgeon less material to work with. Cartilage can be transferred (such as an ear or rib graft), but it requires a great deal of effort and skill to sculpt the nose in a natural manner.

The nose is an organ with very special functions, not just an aesthetic feature. It also assists with breathing, immunity, balance, and even sensory awareness. If the original plastic surgery impaired basic nose function, so that you have trouble breathing, cannot smell, or face similar issues, the revision procedure becomes increasingly complicated. When possible, I always attempt to improve both nasal function as well as cosmetic appearance, but previous damage may prevent full restoration of function and cosmetic appearance.

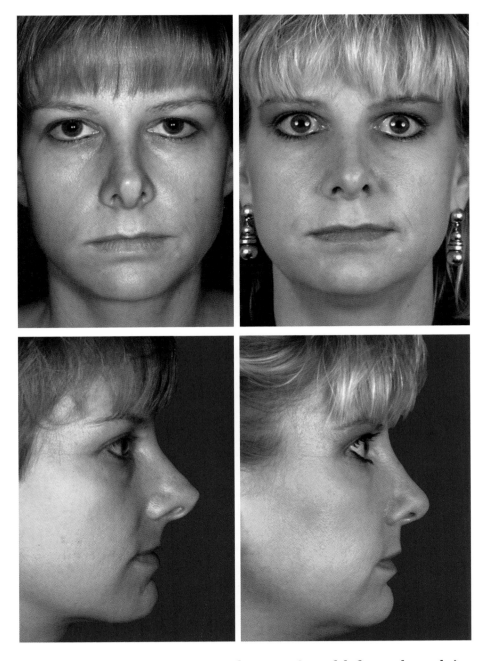

Revision rhinoplasty patient with correction of deformed nasal tip. Significant improvement post-op with a natural appearing nose.

Taking all this into consideration, begin with an in-depth consultation with an expert rhinoplasty surgeon, who can assess what can and what cannot be done. **As with other complex surgeries, decide what three changes are most important to you in order to restore your nose's appearance and function. Make sure these desires are realistic and focus on these priorities first. You've had enough grief with your first surgery, so concentrate on clear communication this second time around.**

Beware of unscrupulous "surgeons" who want to perform multiple revision surgeries in quick succession—this should be an instant red flag. I recently had a patient who had undergone five nasal surgeries on her nose in the preceding three years. That's beyond excessive! Why? Because you must allow the nasal area to heal before your next surgery or scar induces scar. Any major nose revisions should be performed at least twelve to eighteen months apart, allowing the nose and facial area to fully heal. It takes that long for your first procedure to mature into its final state. There is generally no good reason for any doctor to be treating you sooner.

That same patient needed a long treatment process. In order to restore her nasal function and appearance, we needed time to work with natural wound healing. Twelve months after her initial consult, she came back to see me, now showing substantial scar tissue formation in the nose and severe hardening. I waited another six months, during which her nose softened, and I corrected her significant nasal deformity.

A surgeon can temporarily use fillers to restore some of a patient's nasal shape and facial contouring during the waiting period after surgery, but this is limited in terms of results and always temporary.

You can best avoid being a victim by finding a true expert rhinoplasty surgeon initially. As all medical procedures entail risk, not even the best surgeon can guarantee his or her results.

Secondary Face and Neck Lift

The most common issue I see with facelift patients is taut, pulled skin and a windswept look. Many patients had undergone the harsher style of facelift that was done in the eighties and nineties before facial rejuvenation techniques (which focus on adding lost volume rather than just pulling the skin and deep layers tight over the remaining layers) became the norm. These types of procedures were routine at the time. Facelifts done in this manner do not look natural because they do not address the underlying cause of facial aging: loss of facial fat (fullness). Secondary facelift patients often need a combination of "The Five R's" to provide for a more natural facial rejuvenation:

- **R**esect the old scar tissue

- **R**elease the deep scar tissue in the mid-face

- **R**efill the deep fat compartments to soften the face

- **R**eshape the face and neck by reshaping the skin and deep layers

- **R**estore your face to the appearance of an un-operated, youthful face

The goal of these procedures is to restore the patient to a normal non-operative appearance in which no one can tell they have had work done. In patients who have undergone overly aggressive facelifts, this will require a balance of filling in the volume (from depleted fat compartments) that should have been restored in the primary facelift, and giving special consideration to any damage done in their first surgery, such as too much skin removed.

When too much skin is removed in the primary procedure, the patient requires a greater degree of revision. Patients must understand the risks and limitations of what can and cannot be done for them in follow-up surgeries. The procedure is significantly more challenging than a primary procedure. The results can be limited because of previous scarring (which cannot always be cleaned up) and insufficient fat tissue and skin.

Frequently, I see examples of overdone facelift surgeries and I cannot help feeling bad for these people. Poorly done plastic surgery is very

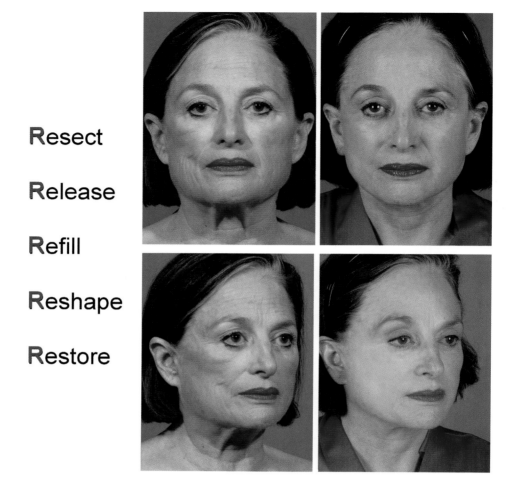

Resect

Release

Refill

Reshape

Restore

Secondary facelift patient after a "Lift and Fill" facelift with the 5 R's to provide for a more natural facial rejuvenation

noticeable and really can be avoided with the choice of a good plastic surgeon. One common excuse is with price. I hear people say, "A procedure is the same anywhere you get it and this surgeon's prices are lower." That kind of strategy would be fine for the purchase of a widescreen TV or a sofa, but certainly not for face or body-improvement surgery. And no, a procedure is not just a procedure. Each person's procedure requires a completely special, personalized result. Choose wisely the first time and treat yourself with respect.

A very dear friend of mine had a series of procedures done, including a facelift. She expressed the idea of wanting another one, as it had been ten years since her first one. I was extremely concerned, as she is beautiful but had an obvious "too tight" look to her. I sent her to Dr. Rohrich for a consult regarding facial rejuvenation. Today, not only is the windswept look gone, but she has a far more youthful and restored look to her beauty. So the lesson here is the same: get the right revision plastic surgeon.

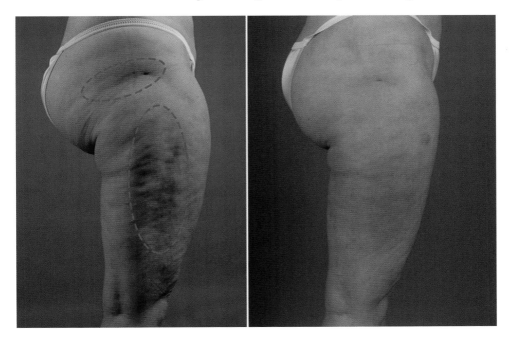

Circled areas where too much fat was removed in previous liposuction surgery (Overdone liposuction is commonly seen)

Secondary Liposuction and Body Contouring

The primary causes of complications in secondary body-contouring patients are similar to those in facelift patients: too much fat or skin removed. However, the body tends to be slightly more forgiving than the face when pulling the skin too tight. We don't lose fat in our bodies as we age the way we do in our faces. The greater risk is actually over-resection (removal) of fat, which can result in severe contour depressions.

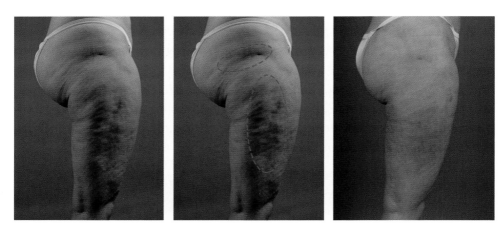

Severe thigh contour deformity corrected by secondary body contouring with fat re-injection into these areas

In some cases, particularly in liposuction surgery, over-resection is immediately apparent once swelling subsides. In other cases, unnatural distribution of body fat can be the result of gaining or losing weight after the surgery—this is why it is so important to reach close to your ideal weight before reshaping and to maintain that weight with diet and exercise after your procedure. If your depressions are a result of weight gain, I recommend that you try to lose the weight before having a secondary procedure.

Fat transfers provide an excellent remedy for depleted fat deposits or contour depressions. While fat is much easier to harvest and transfer than cartilage, redoing overly aggressive liposuction is still quite challenging. Revision surgeries are always difficult, and you may require one to two operative procedures.

In a previous surgery, this liposuction patient had too much fat removed from challenging areas causing depression deformities.

The best remedy is *prevention*. Speak openly with your surgeon before the first surgery, and understand that liposuction does not remove massive amounts of fat, but simply sculpts fat deposits. Remember, it is *far* easier to go back and remove a little more than to try and replace what has been removed—it is therefore best if your surgeon is conservative and errs on the side of caution in performing liposuction.

The other common issue I see with excisional body contouring surgery is highly visible scars that are misplaced or have widened.

Properly placed scars will be mostly concealed in the natural contours of your body, but I often see scars that don't fall where they should. This can happen when the incision is made in the wrong place or if the scar migrates because of significant weight change. Weight gain can also cause scars to widen. If your scars have moved or widened in this way, make the effort to lose weight before revision surgery, as scars can shift and change with each substantial fluctuation in weight.

Secondary Breast Enhancement

The major issues I see in patients dissatisfied with their breast enhancements are implant sizes that are out of proportion with the body, breast asymmetry, implant hardness, and severe scarring. A secondary procedure can address these issues, but, as always, prevention is the wisest strategy. The previously mentioned issues can be avoided by performing breast work that is suitable for each individual patient.

Implant hardness and the use of implants that are too large are the most common causes of complications in breast augmentation. There are limitations on how much you can increase breast size, such as a patient's chest diameter, the amount of breast tissue, and the characteristics of the skin envelope around her breast.

Most female breasts have some degree of asymmetry, whether it is readily noticeable to the eye or not. You really need a plastic surgeon with expertise in breast surgery who can spot and assess preexisting asymmetries pre-op as they are amplified when not corrected at the initial procedure. This is especially true the more bra cup sizes you step up. An experienced breast plastic surgeon will be able to assess exactly what is the optimal size implant for your body.

Implant hardness, one of the most common complications of breast augmentation, is usually caused by capsular contracture. Too much scar tissue forms around the implant and begins to squeeze, resulting in hardness, misshapen appearance, and sometimes, pain. A certain amount of scar tissue around the implant is normal and a good thing—it holds the implant in place—but too much built up over time is definitely a problem.

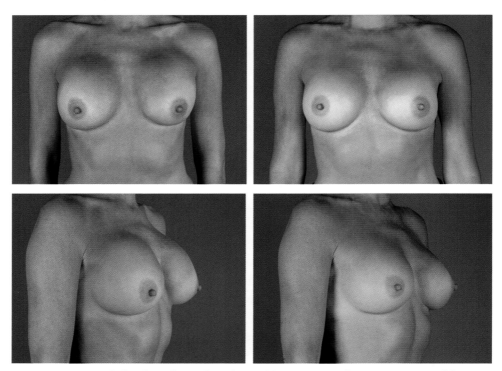

Patient with high riding, hardened breast implants corrected by capsule removal and implant replacement

Revision surgery for hardened implants involves removing the implant and scar tissue and replacing the implant. Your surgeon needs to assess the reason for hardening and try to remedy the problem during the secondary surgery. The implant should be placed below the muscle of the chest wall in most revision surgeries, if it wasn't done this way initially. I almost always place the implant below the muscle the first time, which makes the breast look more natural, as not doing so increases the risk of implant hardening. A textured implant placed under the muscle provides the lowest possible risk of recurrent hardness in the long term. In some severe cases, one may even need to add fat underneath the skin to improve the overall result.

One of the most common complaints with patients undergoing a secondary breast lift is excessive scarring. The scar should be hidden in the breast fold as much as possible, but know that it will sometimes be visible. Some scarring is to be expected. **Genetics determine 90 percent of how a patient heals and the other 10 percent is your surgeon.**

Most incision scars can be hardened and red for six to twelve months, possibly longer in patients who are young, have darker skin tones, or a history of scarring or keloids (irregular fibrous tissue formed at the site of a scar).

All plastic surgery procedures, especially revision surgery, require a tradeoff, and in the case of secondary breast lifts, the tradeoff often includes scarring in order to achieve improved shape and volume.

Closing Thoughts—Don't Be Discouraged, Secondary Surgery Works if…

As you have probably noticed, much of this has been an overview of the limitations and potential difficulties of undergoing cosmetic surgery that has not been done right the first time. **Before engaging in a secondary surgery, both the patient and the plastic surgeon must be prepared and honest about what can and—most importantly—cannot be done.** With these limitations in mind, you can expect to see some marked improvement following a secondary procedure.

Five Key Points to Remember:

1. Secondary surgeries fall into three categories:

    a. Gravitational changes and aging after the primary or first surgery

    b. Complications from the primary surgery

    c. Surgery not done well the first time

2. Secondary surgeries are usually more complex and involved, so you need a "true plastic surgery expert." Ask the **Three Magic Questions** and you will save so much grief, time, and money.

3. Patients need to research and be diligent in finding the best plastic surgeon who has the expertise needed for secondary procedures.

4. Be realistic regarding your overall goals and limit them to your top three! Speak openly with your surgeon and listen well.

5. The goal is for the patient to clearly understand **what can or cannot be done when having secondary or revision surgery procedures.**

Getting Ready for Your Surgery:
How to Make It Easy on Yourself

11

You've done your homework. You've decided on the procedure or procedures that would most enhance your beauty and your self-image. You've worked hard to identify and meet with the right plastic surgeon whose training, prior experience, and rapport all match up with your needs and requirements—a true expert for the procedure(s) you want done.

If you continue now to prepare properly for this important and transformative day, you can proceed much more relaxed and confident. Let this chapter serve as the basis for a final checklist of the things you need to have completed before your surgery date.

ARE ALL OF YOUR QUESTIONS ANSWERED?

Make a list of any questions or concerns you still have. **It is a good idea to cross-reference this list with the one you compiled for your initial consultation. Is there anything you forgot to ask or is still unclear? If the answer is yes, call or make one more appointment before your surgery date.**

Something I have heard voiced by other patients over and over is their hesitation to ask questions. This is all about you and there is no need to feel this way. As patients, we sometimes feel like we don't want to "pester" our surgeon. Don't fall into this category. I was never afraid to ask a question. A great surgeon such as Dr. Rohrich will want you to know all the answers to any concerns you may have. Your surgeon wants to put you at ease with your procedure. **As a patient, you have a right and a duty to feel comfortable and be fully informed. Make sure you have your surgical companion on board to help you pre-op and post-op. This person will be invaluable to you for positive and supportive assistance through this process.**

Are You Clear About All Surgical Fees?

You will receive a complete breakdown of fees from your surgeon's office. This is not a quote but a detailed explanation of all charges specific to your particular procedure or procedures, including fees for the operating room, your surgeon, and anesthesia.

Billing is a straightforward process, but it shouldn't be your focus on the day of your procedure. Be sure to take care of financial matters in advance.

Are All of Your Lab Work and Consent Forms Completed?

All necessary lab work needs to be completed and cleared with your surgeon well before your surgery day. Some of these tests may take time to process, so make sure you have done them in the correct time frame as set out by your surgeon's office. **You also need to complete, sign, and return all necessary paperwork to your plastic surgeon's office, including your pre-op informed consent form. This form is very important and states that you understand all details and any risks related to your procedure to which you have consented.**

These documents can be somewhat tedious and technical, but you must read your paperwork, especially the pre-op consent form, carefully! If there's something you don't fully understand, ask your plastic surgeon or someone at your surgeon's office for clarification.

The pre-op consent form deserves special attention. It is an agreement between you and your surgeon, and you should treat it as an overview of what your surgeon will perform. Remember, this form must state all possible, though not probable, risks and complications. Don't get all worked up about this since it is a list of every complication ever reported. Have you ever read the warning label on aspirin? If you did, you probably would be more hesitant to take it.

Have You Obtained Preoperative Medical Clearance if Necessary?

Preoperative medical clearance simply means that you have been fully evaluated and determined to be a good candidate for your procedure. This requires that you fully disclose all relevant medical history. **And remember: no smoking for four to six weeks leading up to (and after) your procedure. Smoking increases your risk and complication rate significantly. I always remind my residents and fellow plastic surgeons that we are all medical doctors first and foremost and then plastic surgeons second. We always live by the Hippocratic Oath—*First do no harm!***

Disclose everything to your surgeon. Be sure to reveal in full any underlying medical conditions to your surgeon—diabetes, hypertension, and allergies, *anything* you have been diagnosed with. *It is absolutely mandatory* that you discuss them with your surgeon so they can assess your risk of complications from a fully informed position. Many minor ailments may not affect your surgery, but disclose them anyway, for your safety. Don't forget to mention any medications (including over-the-counter) you are taking. **Make sure that your surgeon, your surgery companion, and all members of the medical staff are aware of any allergic reactions you have ever had to any medications. Also, be sure to inform your surgeon about any current or past history of alcohol or substance abuse, as this could affect what medications you can be given safely during your operation and recovery.**

If you are unsure whether or not some fact is relevant, err on the side of caution and disclose the information.

I know a lot of people who have had surgery who sometimes "forget" to mention something to their surgeon—such as a past history of alcoholism or substance abuse. Don't be embarrassed or shy about dis-closing personal information to your surgeon. By now, you should have built a strong rapport and trust. They really do need to be fully informed about your medical history and lifestyle choices. It matters! Some medica-tions you may be given are cross-tolerant with alcohol and other drugs, and you definitely want to take these medications seriously. The last thing you want is to be given a medication that is going to cause you more problems during your recovery from surgery.

*Drugs, alcohol, and medications are not the only things that can in-teract with your surgery medications—many foods and supplements can as well! Be sure to disclose all supplements you are taking, especially the four **G**'s that can cause excessive bleeding after your operation—**G**inger, **G**inseng, **G**arlic, and **G**inkgo biloba. I was shocked when Dr. Rohrich ex-plained that garlic could cause more bruising.*

Did You Select a Surgery Date That Works for You?

Consider the date of your surgery carefully. When setting your date, make sure to allow ample time for both preparation and recovery. You need to allow yourself sufficient time off work and from any other ob-ligations so that you have time to heal before you can return to your normal daily routines.

Below is a list of average recovery times for some of the more common aesthetic plastic surgery procedures:

These time frames are only averages and can vary, of course, but they are safe estimates for the majority of procedures and patients. Talk with your surgeon about the realistic recovery time for your particular procedure. It can be a good idea to set aside a little more time, if possible. It's better to err on the side of caution and take off a few more days than needed than risk having to return to work or other obligations before you are completely ready. Everyone heals slightly differently, so always be pre-pared to take a couple of extra days if needed to recover.

- Rhinoplasty—7–10 days

- Facelift—2 weeks

- Eyelids or brows—10 days

- Laser or chemical peels—12–14 days

- Breast augmentation—5–7 days

- Tummy tuck—2 weeks

- Liposuction—5–7 days

Do You Have Your Surgery Companion With You?

You want someone to serve as a confidante, friend, and personal assistant during your procedure and recovery. **We will refer to this person as your surgery companion, and they should be there for you pre-op, during surgery, and throughout early aftercare, so be sure to get someone you can depend on. A good surgery companion will make your recovery an easier and more pleasant experience. They should be trustworthy, positive, and encouraging.**

Your surgery companion should fully understand your procedure as well as what is expected of them afterwards. Keep them fully informed about all aspects of your procedure and abreast of any changes to the plan. Provide them with a copy of the preoperative and postoperative instructions from your surgeon's office to read ahead of time.

They will drive you to and from your surgery and stay with you once you get home. In the highly unlikely event of an emergency, you want to feel safe knowing you have someone around whom you can trust and depend upon. In my office, we never allow patients to go home by themselves immediately following a procedure. All patients either stay in our hotel, with nursing staff present 24/7, or they are released, if and when appropriate, to the care of a companion. Even if you will be staying in an aftercare facility during the first few days of your recovery, you will still need someone to stay with you at least the first night, and possibly the second.

This is so important! Realize that you are asking a lot of your surgery companion and treat them considerately. Line up your surgery companion well in advance of your surgery day and keep them abreast of any changes to your plans, not only for your sake, but also out of consideration for them.

Choose a companion who knows you well already. They could be a friend, spouse, or family member—anyone who will be helpful, compassionate, caring, and noncritical. What is most important is that, whoever they are, you can trust and depend on them. You want someone who is generally positive and will not be critical of you or your surgery. *They are, after all, in a supportive role and you need them to support you throughout your procedure and recovery.*

A surgery companion provides not only emotional support but also support with the practical matters related to your surgery. They can help with the proper instructions and with administering medications, monitoring your condition, getting you in and out of bed if you need help in the first few days post-op, and being there in case there is a concern or an emergency. As a practical matter, it would help if they were not squeamish. Those who are easily upset by unpleasant sights or situations might not be ideal to have around during the days following your surgery.

Make Sure Your Surgeon and You Are of the Same Mindset Pre-Op

You will want to speak with your surgeon regarding any last-minute questions or concerns directly before your surgery. This is extremely important. **You want to be absolutely sure that you and your surgeon are both on the same page regarding every aspect of your** procedure. I always see my patients in the pre-op area to discuss exactly what we are going to do. This is critical to put the patient at ease immediately pre-op. This is especially true with regard to anesthesia, which we have covered in Chapter 3.

Have You Filled All of Your Prescriptions?

Any medication prescribed by your surgeon should be filled prior to surgery. After your surgery, you are likely to be uncomfortable and perhaps a little groggy from anesthesia and any pain medications. After surgery is not a time for making a run to the pharmacy!

When packing your bags, keep all of the medications your surgeon has prescribed for you together in one place. Make sure your surgery companion knows where these medications are so they can give them to the attending nurse in the aftercare facility. The nursing staff will administer all medications while you are in the aftercare facility as well as all other medications you take on a daily basis. Once you return home as an outpatient, your surgery companion should take this duty over until you feel up to managing it yourself.

Don't forget to purchase an over-the-counter stool softener like MiraLAX®, which is excellent to prevent post-op constipation caused by taking your pain medications like codeine.

In addition to filling all of the prescriptions prescribed by your surgeon before going in for surgery, also pick up any prescriptions or over-the-counter medications you take regularly. Be sure you have enough of all of your medications to last the first week. You don't want to run out of an important medication while you are still recovering. It's just easier to have everything ready and in place.

Again, be very careful about mixing medications without first informing your surgeon—over-the-counter medications and herbal supplements are medicines, too, and they count! If there's any doubt, tell your surgeon before taking anything at all before your procedure or during recovery. Always bring your medications with you on the day of your procedure if you are staying overnight.

Have You Gone Grocery Shopping and Picked Up Household Essentials?

You have medicine covered—but what about food? The last thing most people want to do when they get home from surgery is a big shopping trip. Stock your fridge and freezer before your surgery. You want to have plenty of easily digestible food on hand such as applesauce, yogurt, broths, puddings, Jell-O, or crackers, especially during the first few days after your surgery. Many medications, including pain medications, should be taken with food.

Talk to your surgeon about what foods are appropriate. In general, avoid spicy and salty foods. Spicy foods can upset your stomach, and salt causes fluid retention. **In the initial days and weeks of your recovery period, maintain a diet that is both low in sodium and high in protein, as this will allow for optimal wound healing.**

Ask your surgeon when you can return to a normal, well-balanced diet. Remember, a diet high in lean protein is going to help with tissue repair and recovery. You will be back to your normal routine in no time so don't let yourself feel rushed. Enjoy this time off and focus on the beauty of your transformation process.

In addition to food and medication, make sure you have any other personal items you may need, such as toiletries and reading and viewing materials. Make sure you have clean clothes, clean sheets, and everything ready to go—these may seem like small things, but they can be quite comforting when you are in recovery.

Don't worry too much about preparation—if you forget something, you can always have your surgery companion run to the store for you, throw a load of clothes in the laundry, or do any small things you forgot to do. Just make it easy as you can and take care of yourself.

Do You Have Ice and Ice Packs On Hand?

Cold compresses or cold gelatin masks (such as Swiss Therapy™ eye masks) can work wonders when it comes to reducing swelling and bruising for the first few days, especially during the first 72 hours. They are especially necessary if you are doing your eyes or having any kind of facial surgery. Your surgeon's office will provide you with eye masks or you can also use crushed ice in small plastic bags, which work well, too. You want at least two ice packs so you can always keep at least one on ice, fresh and cold. Your surgeon should have them on hand, so ask for an extra.

Ice packs are especially important for those having surgery of the face, as facial swelling can be particularly bothersome and pronounced, but they are just as helpful for reducing swelling and pain in other areas as well. Have them on hand no matter what procedure you are having, just in case.

Keep in mind that ice packs and ice compresses should not be left directly on the skin continually, no matter how good they may feel—rotate them on and off every 20 minutes to avoid excessive cold on the skin, which can be damaging to the tissue. Keep this up for the first five days post-op.

In a pinch, keep several bags of frozen peas or rice in your freezer to change them out, as they will work just as well as an ice pack if you find yourself without one. Don't forget to stretch lightly but do not bend over if you had a rhinoplasty or facial cosmetic surgery, and get up, move, and take walks. This really helps.

Know What to Avoid After Your Surgery— And Know It Before Your Surgery

The following are things you will probably want to consider cutting out of your life while you are in recovery. Avoid all of the following:

- **Negative people**—They suck the life out of you, and you can't afford that when you're recuperating! Avoid those who are not empathetic or those who are critical about your surgery or surgical goals. While it is great that such people care about you, chances are they do not understand plastic surgery and may have inaccurate or irrational views of your procedure. Cut such negative forces out of your life during this critical time. You will have enough to focus on as it is. **At the same time, try to surround your-self with positive and supportive people you trust, such as a wonderful and supportive surgery companion, who helps alleviate some of your uncertainty, anxieties, and loneliness during the process.**

- **Alcohol**—It can cause bleeding, slow healing, and interact with medications. This is very important—do not mix alcohol with your medications, especially your pain medications. Do not drink alcohol within 24 hours of taking any pain or anxiety medications.

- **Smoking and smokers**—Absolutely no smoking for at least four weeks pre- and post-op! Avoid secondhand smoke as well.

Packing Your Surgery Bag—What Do You Need to Bring?

When it comes to packing your bags for your surgery day, you want to be careful to take everything you need, but only what you need. Keep it simple. You don't want to forget necessities, nor do you want to have to keep track of excess items you won't use. A good surgery companion will come in handy here—they can help assemble and keep track of your items. You'll need the following:

- All of your **prescribed medications.** (Pain medications, anti-anxiety medications, antibiotics, if needed.)

- **A couple of pairs of button-down or open-front pajamas** depending on how long you will be staying in the aftercare facility. They must be button-down or open-front as you will not be able to or want to put anything over your head while you heal.

- Your own non-slip **slippers**.

- **Toiletries** including facial wash, a toothbrush, lip balm, etc. Be sure you clear things like facial washes with your surgeon before applying them to any area of your body in which you have had surgery. **Forget makeup—you won't need it.**

- **Appropriate clothes for going home.** You want comfortable clothing to wear home that is easy to put on and doesn't require going over your head, such as a button-down shirt or zip-up jacket or shirt. Bring comfortable pants and shoes as well.

I would also suggest sharing your list of items to pack with your surgeon's office or surgical companion. They might be able to point out something you are forgetting as well as items that you won't really need.

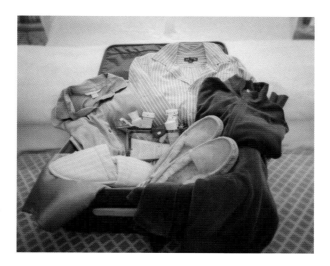

Getting ready – simple items to take with you

Five Key Points to Remember:

1. **Know before you go**—You want to be fully prepared before the day of your procedure. If you still have further concerns or questions regarding your procedure, call or make an appointment well before your surgery date. Trust your selected plastic surgeon—you did your homework, now let the plastic surgeon do his or her work for you.

2. **Arrange to have your surgery companion ready** to be with you both on the day of your surgery and during your postoperative recovery.

3. **Take the right amount of time off from work and other obligations**—plus a few days more, just in case.

4. **Have all your postoperative medications and regular medications** that you have cleared with your surgeon (diabetes, allergy, and hypertension medications, for example) ready and together. Prepare your home in advance: have your groceries and other items on hand, including anything you need for your particular procedure, such as a pillow wedge after having a facelift.

5. **Get out of bed with the help of your nursing staff and/or your surgical companion and get moving as soon as possible and don't forget to eat healthy (high protein, low salt, plenty of fluids, etc.).** This will set you on the road to recovery.

GETTING READY FOR SURGERY

TEN POINT CHECKLIST

1. Make sure your questions are fully answered.

2. Scheduled time off and surgery date selected

3. Surgery fees clarified and understood

4. All lab work and consent forms completed

5. Surgery companion arranged/informed about procedure(s)

6. Necessary medications stopped (including aspirin)

7. Supplements/medications prescriptions filled (bring them with you)

8. Ice packs on hand

9. Household shopping complete

10. Surgery bag packed

Recovering—Knowing What to Expect, Being Prepared, and Getting Back to Normal

12

Your procedure isn't over when you leave the operating room.

Comprehensive surgical care always includes quality aftercare, and the surgical process isn't over until you have completely recovered. Your surgeon will not be with you once you go home, but should be available if needed. Your part as a patient is to make sure you and your surgery companion understand your aftercare instructions, follow them diligently, and keep your surgeon's office up to date about your status. Keep your surgeon informed by attending all of your post-op visits, knowing what to expect and watch out for, and call your surgeon's office immediately if you have concerns or questions.

Proper aftercare is critical to good outcomes—make sure you take care of the area operated upon in order to minimize scarring and protect the work your surgeon has done. Yet many patients don't think about aftercare until it is already upon them. Don't make this mistake. Realize that what happens during your recovery is just as important as what happens in the operating room. The difference is that the onus is now on you to manage more of your own care.

By the end of this chapter, you should be well informed about the basics of aftercare and better prepared to face your recovery process confidently.

Suddenly faced with the prospect of going home alone, you may feel bewildered. Many patients even find going home after their surgery frightening or discomforting. This is normal as you have been under the direct care and supervision of your plastic surgeon and surgery team.

*Realize that you're not alone. **For one, you have your surgery companion whom you can depend upon and trust. Hopefully, you also have a wide network of supportive and positive friends and family.** You also have the advice, companionship, and guidance Dr. Rohrich and I are offering through this book. Finally, do not forget that you still have your plastic surgeon and their office to draw upon for support, reassurance, and care. Your outstanding plastic surgeon should follow you through recovery long term.*

We hope we have helped you reach the very important decisions, clear up any confusion, and have touched on any questions or anxieties you may have had before reading this book. This is especially critical in the first few weeks after your surgery, when you will still be healing, but no longer under the constant care of your surgery team.

Your Aftercare Instructions (Overview)

Here are some points that will guide you through what to do—and what not to do—when you return home after your surgery. These are concerns and considerations common to most, if not all, surgeries:

- **First and foremost, follow your surgeon's post-op instructions.** The individualized advice and instruction of your own quality surgeon always supersedes whatever else you hear from friends, family, and other nonprofessional opinions. Make sure you have a copy of the instructions from your surgeon's office. These are custom-tailored for your procedure and individualized for your situation.

- **Get plenty of rest.** What is recovery for, if not ample rest and relaxation? It's time to veg out a little and take some "me time." Just make sure you're paying close attention to your progress and condition. Don't disregard anything!

- **Get moving as quickly as possible.** Despite the need to take time for rest throughout your recovery, you also need to get up and moving as soon as possible. This will help with circulation, expedite the healing process, and lower the risk for blood clots. While in bed, be sure to flex your ankles often. When it comes to moving around, you should start slowly. In the first few days following your surgery, it is enough to take brief walks for a few minutes at a time. Increase the duration of these walks gradually over time, being careful to listen to both your surgeon's instructions and what your body is telling you.

- **Do not exercise for the first three to four weeks.** While you do want to get moving right away, you do not want to start exercising too soon as this can actually hamper your recovery. Remember to keep your heart rate below 100 beats per minute for the first three to four weeks. In the fourth week, you normally can resume most of your exercise and workouts, but please clear with your surgeon first.

- **Remember that healing varies from patient to patient.** Recovery is, at its heart, the process of healing. It can be very easy to get caught up in expectations. Remember that the guidelines laid out in this book are just based on the averages we have seen, but it can, and will, vary. **Do not get worried if you take longer to heal than someone you know or the average time—read that, average time—listed in this book. Recovery is brief and your results are forever, so try not to get hung up on or depressed if you take a little longer than most. It's not worth the stress.**

- **Avoid sex early post-op.** You should completely avoid sex for two to three weeks in most cases. Depending on the details of your surgery, this may be shorter or longer. In many cases, it may be a good idea to limit sexual activities to those that are passive or involve limited movement for the first month or more. Do not be embarrassed to discuss this with your surgeon.

- **Watch for signs of early post-op depression.** Some patients suffer from mild depression after surgery—this is not uncommon. It can be due to anxiety over your surgery and outcome, the stress of the healing process, or any number of factors. Whatever the cause, do watch out for these common signs of depression following surgery (it is normal to feel somewhat depressed or "down" early post-op up to two to three weeks):

- Feeling inexplicably sad, down, or disengaged

- Appetite loss

- Insomnia

- Inability to return to daily routines even after fully healing

- Difficulty concentrating

Anesthesia and prescription medications used in surgery and aftercare can also contribute to feelings of depression and may further exacerbate difficulties with concentration. These side effects should be short-lived, but if they are not, speak with your surgeon and, when appropriate, a mental health professional. There are medications and treatments that can help.

Feeling depressed post-op is a frequent occurrence, and I have seen it among my friends who have had surgery. Though usually mild, this depression can still be quite detrimental to quality of life in the short term. Understand that it is normal to have some feelings of sadness or apprehension after such a major event as surgery, but these feelings generally pass within a few days. If they do not, or if you think you may be experiencing severe or major depression, you may want to consult your plastic surgeon about finding a qualified mental health provider. Generally, these feelings are mild and transient and can be worked through with short-term medication. Depression and anxiety are not things you should fear or allow to deter you from your surgery goals.

- **Learn to depend on your surgery companion.** This is very important, because this is the person whom you picked to see you through your surgery. After your surgery, you will probably feel weak and drowsy from the anesthesia and operation. You may require help getting in and out of bed the first few times. **You really want to have someone around to stay with you for the first 24 to 48 hours. Depending upon your procedure, your surgery companion's assistance could be very helpful for the first week or so.**

All of my friends who have had surgery have said the same thing. ***When they talk about their surgery companion, the thing they say time and time again is: "They had me." So now you have this book, and you want to have a "me" as a trusted and knowledgeable person you can count on throughout your recovery. A good surgery companion can go a long way toward making your journey as easy as possible.*** *In addition, our book will help navigate you to a seamless recovery.*

- **Expect and accept swelling—it is temporary.** Swelling varies from patient to patient—this is just another part of the healing process. Resolution of swelling is a large part of recovery. In fact, you should not consider your outcome complete until after swelling has resolved. If you are concerned, seek your surgeon's assurance.

- **Elevate areas of your body that have been operated upon.** While swelling is inevitable, there are things you can do to minimize it. Keeping operated-upon areas elevated prevents fluid from building, which substantially decreases swelling. Use pillows and/or a wedge rest as appropriate, especially when sleeping.

- **Remember to eat right.** It can be easy to forget to eat well—or even at all—after your surgery. **Protein** is important for tissue and cell repair, and a high protein diet will facilitate a quick recovery. You may, however, have to follow a restricted diet for the first few days. You may need to eat foods that are easy to digest or easy to chew such as broths, applesauce, yogurt, gelatin snacks, and similar easily digestible foods. Talk to your surgeon about what is and is not acceptable to eat and when you can return to your normal healthy diet. Consider using a stool softener as well so you don't have to strain when using the restroom after your procedure—straining can put stress on sutures.

- **Do not fly immediately after your surgery.** Doing so can cause excessive swelling. Most patients can fly after ten to twelve days, but you need to get approval from your plastic surgeon before doing so. Not being able to fly can be especially problematic for patients who are traveling out of town to see a surgeon. You may need to find another means of travel. Obviously, it's best to plan for this in advance.

- **Take your pain medication as prescribed.** You may not need pain medication, depending on your procedure and your tolerance for discomfort, but if you do, take it only as prescribed. Remember to never ever consume alcohol with pain or anxiety medications and to speak with your surgeon about any other drugs you are taking.

- **Alert your surgeon if you have a history of alcohol or substance abuse.** This is extremely important; please do not disregard it. If you have a history of alcoholism or substance abuse, it is absolutely mandatory that you discuss this with your plastic surgeon.

I have seen some of my friends and patients alike struggle with this. Realize these are powerful medications you are taking. Most people have no problem with medications as long as they are taken as prescribed, but some do have problems. Be honest with yourself and your surgeon. Being open to discussion regarding any and all medications will help make your recovery easier.

Be aware of the signs of infection. Some of the most common symptoms of infection are the following:

- Increased pain or a fever of 101 degrees Fahrenheit or above

- If you are suddenly exhausted or lethargic (This is different from patients feeling tired after anesthesia from surgery, which tends to get better with each day.)

- If an incision begins to feel hot to the touch or abnormally red, swollen, or has foul-smelling drainage

If any one of these situations arises, contact your surgeon or surgeon's office immediately.

Take care of your incisions. Be sure you are clear on how to take care of your incisions both before and after any staples or sutures are removed. Your surgeon will provide you with instructions regarding care for all incisions and treatment for scars. You may want or need to use scar cream—be sure to seek your surgeon's advice before applying any product to the operated area. **(Please see the wound care sheet and incision aftercare timeline at the end of this chapter for detailed guidelines.)**

Dr. Rohrich obviously cannot address those considerations that are particular to your individual aftercare. We simply cannot know all of the idiosyncrasies of your situation and the particulars of your procedure. No matter how thorough this book may be, we cannot provide you with the comprehensive and individualized care of your own qualified surgeon.

Facelifts and Neck Lifts

- Keep your head elevated at a 45-degree angle for the first two weeks using a wedge rest or well-placed pillow.

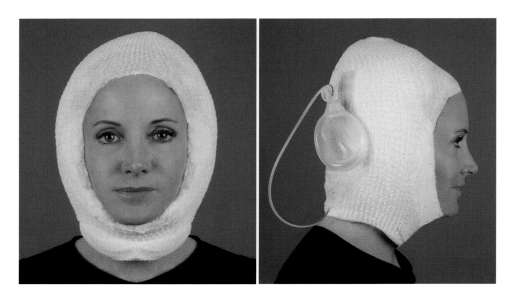

Facelift wrap with drain in place

- Any head wrappings and bandages are usually removed after 48 hours, though this can vary from surgeon to surgeon and procedure to procedure.

  This is so true and a huge sense of relief. This will allow you to feel somewhat more normal again. It's the first major step in recovery and is (quite literally!) a liberating feeling to unwrap. Please know that nothing about the head wrapping or bandages is painful. There is no real pain in the face after a facelift, but sutures and staples can be annoying more than anything.

- **Apply light ice packs or Swiss Therapy™ eye masks to the exposed areas of the face to reduce swelling.** This is especially critical for the first 72 hours after your surgery, but can be continued for as long as necessary. Ice packs need to be kept cold, so it is good to keep at least two so you can rotate them so that you always have a fresh one in the freezer.

- **Dressing and drains are normally removed within the first few days.** Your surgeon will provide instructions on how to care for them—until then, be sure to share this and all information with your surgery companion. Whatever you do, do not pull on or

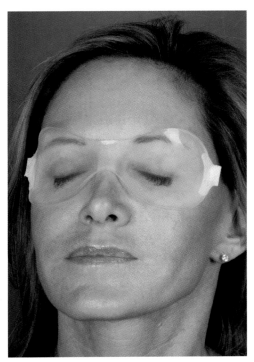

Gel eye mask used to minimize postoperative bruising and swelling

remove your own drains! You will notice suture tightening during healing, which can be uncomfortable, but is normal. If you have any staples, these may also be uncomfortable. The tightening is actually a good sign of healing. Both are usually removed within seven to ten days.

- **Your hair should be washed for you in the aftercare facility before you go home after your dressing and drains are removed.** At this point you can begin shampooing at home with a mild shampoo, such as baby shampoo. If you blow dry your hair, use the low and cool settings on your blow dryer. Do not use any hair coloring products for the first three weeks after surgery—you want to give the incisions time to heal first.

- **Swelling of the face is totally normal and occurs in 100 percent of patients.** The degree of swelling varies from patient to patient. All swelling takes time to subside, especially with a lower facelift, but you should see steady progress over the course of days, weeks, and months. Topical arnica gel and bromelain, which are natural extracts, can be immensely helpful in reducing bruising, especially around the neck.

Much of the swelling subsides quickly, and so you will see rapid improvement early on, which is a good thing for certain. Be sure to keep perspective and not get discouraged as progress slows. Lingering swelling will also improve with time. Keeping a journal of your progress can be a good way to keep yourself motivated and your spirits up because you'll have physical proof of your progress. I had a friend who did this with daily photos. It was truly amazing to see the actual healing process with each passing day.

- **You may experience slight asymmetrical swelling, where swelling is uneven on one side of the face or under the chin and around the neck**. This will even out, but it does take time, so don't be alarmed if you still feel or look slightly bumpy (especially in the neck area) after a few weeks. If, however, you notice **extreme swelling**, especially in the beginning, that is far more pronounced on one side of the face, contact your surgeon's office immediately.

- **The majority of patients experience some bruising in the lower face and neck area.** This is completely normal and will go away. Numbness is also common. While numbness will eventually go away as well, it may linger in some areas, such as the sides of face and around the ears, for months or even up to a year.

- **Use sunscreen! You should be doing this already—sun damage is a major cause of facial aging.** You want a sunscreen that is effective at blocking both UVA and UVB rays and that has an SPF of 30 or higher. Furthermore, avoid excessive exposure to sunlight for at least the first eight weeks.

- **Do not smoke.** Not only does smoking accelerate facial aging, it also interferes with the recovery process significantly.

Rhinoplasty

- **Keep your head elevated for the first seven days, including while you're sleeping.** Strategically placed pillows or a wedge type pillow behind your head can help with this.

- **After your surgery, you will have some combination of internal and/or external splints, but no nasal packing.** These are applied in order to support and protect your new nose. These are usually removed after seven to ten days. Do not tamper with these on your own.

- **Do not wear glasses or anything that rests upon the nose for four weeks.** Either use contacts or tape your glasses to your face, as per your surgeon's instructions. You also need to keep the nose protected during any physical injury for the first six months, especially the first month when it is still "soft" and most vulnerable—it is best to avoid any activity that could result in damage to the nose throughout your recovery.

- **As with all surgeries, you will experience swelling, but it can be particularly bothersome to experience swelling of the nose.** The worst swelling will be in the first 72 hours after your surgery. During this time, you should apply crushed ice packs or Swiss Thereapy™ eye pads (obtained from the hospital) to minimize swelling and bruising. Be careful not to put pressure on the nasal splint while doing this.

- **While swelling will reach its peak after 48 to 72 hours, you will have residual nose swelling for weeks or even months.** This is very normal. Very minor residual swelling can linger for up to fifteen months—for this reason, your results will not fully refine and finalize for a year or more. However, your nose will continue to improve in appearance throughout your recovery.

- **All of the general care advice about starting with a light diet applies here as well, but you want to also be careful not to eat anything that requires excessive lip movement, such as apples and corn-on-the-cob, for the first two weeks.**

- You will probably experience a slightly bloody nasal discharge for three to four days. Do not rub, blot, or blow your nose, as this will tend to irritate the area. Instead, use a drip pad under your nose, changing it out as often as needed. You may discard the drip pad and remove the tape on your cheeks once the drainage has stopped. To prevent bleeding, do not blow your nose for the first two weeks after surgery. Try not to sneeze, but if you do, sneeze through your mouth.

  I said it in the chapter on surgery of the nose, but I will say it again here—embrace a little messiness. You just had surgery; you don't need to be a beauty queen right away.

- While the nasal splint is still on, you may have your hair washed in a "salon" style fashion. Take care to prevent the nasal splint from getting wet.

- Keep the inside edges of your nostrils and any stitches clean by using a cotton swab saturated with hydrogen peroxide followed by a thin coating of an anti-bacterial ointment. This will help prevent crust from forming. You will not hurt anything inside your nose as long as you are gentle, and do not insert the cotton swab into your nose further than the cotton tip. (You can stop this after four days.)

Breast Enhancement

- **After surgery, it is important to get out of bed and get moving periodically as soon as you can in order to prevent post-operative problems.** However, do keep movements of the arms to a minimum during the first 48 hours. Do not use your arms to support your body or lift anything heavy, as this will put excessive strain on the operative area.

- **You may have small drains which are used to prevent fluid accumulation (only for breast lifts/reduction/breast explant and replacement).** Make sure you record the output as drains are removed if the drainage is less than 30–40 cc per day. You can usually get back to daily routines quickly, resuming light daily activities after a day or two. Driving may normally be resumed after a week.

- **Maintain a light diet the first day.** You may return to eating normally on the second day.

- **You can shower for the first time 24 hours after your surgery, being careful not to disturb your incisions.**

- **Avoid strenuous exercise for four full weeks, as with other operative procedures.**

- **Do not wear an underwire bra until your surgeon says it is safe—usually this is about six weeks after your surgery.** You may be provided with a specialized support bra, or instructed to wear a camisole or no bra at all.

- **Do not smoke.**

- **It is very important that you begin a routine of breast implant massage starting three to five days after surgery—these are breast exercises that help to prevent breast hardening and capsular contractures.** Someone from your surgery office can explain how to perform these exercises. Commit to doing these exercises on each breast three times daily.

Body Contouring

Generally speaking, the main things to consider after having any body contouring are the general guidelines applicable to all surgeries and proper wound care, since body contouring (with the exception of liposuction-only procedures) involves your surgeon making incisions. Review the section on wound care extra carefully.

- **Recovery time will vary based upon your specific procedure and the area upon which you are operating**—tummy tucks, for example, can have a longer-than-average recovery time.

- **Swelling and fluid retention are normal after body contouring. It takes about four to six weeks,** sometimes longer, for swelling and any fluid retention to fully dissipate. Drains may be placed under the skin to help drain fluid—these will be removed within a few days. Do not pull on any drains or remove them yourself.

In most cases, you can resume most normal routines in about three to four weeks.

Tummy Tuck

Tummy tucks are another type of body contouring, but you do want to take special considerations when recovering from abdominoplasty. Aftercare for abdominoplasty is similar to other body contouring procedures, but can be slightly longer and more complicated due to the area of the operation. Here are some things to keep in mind during recovery:

- **Get up and walk around periodically as soon as possible in order to prevent postoperative problems.** It is good to walk for 15 to 20 minutes six times per day. Try to walk slightly stooped over for the first three to five days to release tension on the suture line.

- **Sleep with your hips in a full flexed position for three to five days.** Keep your head elevated about 30 degrees and leave your knees slightly flexed. When awake, stop to take fifteen to twenty deep breaths each hour to keep your lungs clear.

- **In addition to maintaining a light diet, also avoid spicy food, which can cause nausea and gas.** After two to three days, you may resume a normal high protein diet. Make sure you take a stool softener post-op to prevent constipation.

- **You will need to wear a compression garment continuously for the first seven to ten days.** You may take it off to shower after the first three days—it is best if this is done under the care of your surgeon's office the first time.

- **Your physical activity will be more limited after a tummy tuck relative to most other operations.** Avoid lifting anything over ten pounds for the first three weeks. Do not drive for the first seven days. Abdominal stress on your muscles will stretch or break the sutures if you exercise in the first four weeks—so don't do it! Avoid all sexual activity during this period as well. At that point, you may ease back into exercise and sexual activity slowly, avoiding activities that cause any abdominal movement.

- **Do not take aspirin or products containing aspirin for three weeks after surgery.**

What Dr. Rohrich is saying should not be taken lightly. The extra care he mentions as required during aftercare is because a tummy tuck requires a large incision made in the abdomen in a place that is prone to movement and stretching. Following these guidelines carefully is important to help to minimize the appearance of this scar. Be especially careful about making any movements that put strain on the incision as this can widen the scar. Everyone who undergoes a tummy tuck ends up with a scar, but with proper care of the incision, you can maximize scar healing and minimize the size and appearance of the scar so that it is easily concealed.

Liposuction

- You will have a compression garment on when you wake up in the recovery room. **This must be worn at all times for the first two weeks except to shower daily.** You may remove the garment briefly to shower beginning on the third day of recovery; however, be sure someone, such as a surgery companion, is there to help. You may feel dizzy or light-headed—this is normal, but you want to have someone there to prevent falling. Take your time and rest to regain your balance, if necessary. After the first two weeks, you will need to wear the compression garment at night only for an additional two weeks. You may actually find that the compression garment is more comfortable after your surgery than regular clothing. Many patients continue to wear it beyond the length of time necessary just for comfort's sake. You may also try tight compression garments, and other similar compression garments.

- **Swelling and bruising are normal and can last for as long as three to four months. Itching sensations and numbness in the areas that underwent liposuction are also common—** these will gradually subside over the next two to three months.

- **You may also experience hardness under the skin. Massaging these areas can help alleviate any hardness and improve circulation.** Massage can begin two weeks after surgery and can be performed by yourself or a specialist.

Again, liposuction is not about shedding pounds immediately, but rather about perfecting your body's shape. Once swelling and fluid retention subside, you will see a change, not on the scale, but in the way your clothes fit.

Secondary Surgery

- **Secondary surgeries sometimes have a slightly longer recovery time than primary surgeries because the area has been operated on before.** You may experience more swelling and more bruising as well; however, outcomes are generally favorable.

- **In these (and all) cases, talk to your surgeon about what to expect. The aftercare for your secondary surgery will likely not differ from your primary surgery if corrections need to be made.** For example, your secondary surgery and recovery may be significantly easier than your primary surgery if you are only revising one aspect of your initial procedure.

- **Because secondary surgeries can be more complicated than primary surgeries, you want to be sure that you carefully follow the aftercare instructions you receive precisely to ensure that you see the best possible results.**

Aftercare instructions for secondary surgery are highly dependent upon what procedure you are revising. In general, the procedure and aftercare will be similar to your first surgery since you are having a similar surgery. Though surgery and recovery from secondary procedures are more complicated than primary procedures, you have one great advantage as a secondary patient—the benefit of experience! Take what you learned the first time around and apply it to make your second go-around easier.
    I have compiled an easy ten point checklist for your recovery.

HOW TO MAXIMIZE YOUR RECOVERY

TEN POINT CHECKLIST

1. Keep the operated area elevated above the heart for at least ten days post-op.

2. Eat a high protein/high fiber/low salt diet and drink plenty of fluids.

3. Make sure your surgery companion is available for initial recovery period.

4. Take all medications as needed for pain—keeping ahead of the pain and anxiety. Take antibiotics as prescribed.

5. Keep ice packs on operated areas especially the first three to five days for bruising and swelling—20 minutes on, 20 minutes off.

6. Get up and out of bed often to walk—this improves circulation and prevents blood clots.

7. If you have drains, keep accurate records of drainage.

8. Call your surgeon if you have a fever of 101.5 degrees F. or above, or if you experience unusual increased pain or swelling.

9. No exercise the first three weeks or heart rate above 100. Get clearance to resume a normal exercise routine.

10. No smoking (delays wound healing).

WOUND CARE

Wound care applies to any surgery that requires incisions to be made, including most common aesthetic plastic surgeries. These incisions will heal, mature, refine, and fade substantially over time, but you must take good care of them to ensure proper healing and to prevent infection, excessive scarring, or other complications.

At my office, I hand out the following timeline to my patients, instructing them on how to take care of incisions and other wounds for all the procedures that I perform.

DAYS ONE THROUGH TEN— SEALING/PROTECTING THE SKIN CLOSURE

- Apply an antibiotic ointment sparingly to the suture line for the first two days only. Discontinue ointment after two days as it may cause a skin irritation or reaction (dermatitis). If you have had skin closure with skin glue, you do not need to apply ointment to the area, as it is already sealed.

- You may shower on the first postoperative day. Allow water to hit the area and blot dry. Avoid scrubbing or disturbing the incision.

- Swelling and discoloration usually peak on the third day and then decrease over the next five to seven days.

DAY TEN THROUGH SIX WEEKS: MOLDING /PROTECTING THE SKIN CLOSURE

- All of the remaining skin sutures will be removed if needed by ten to twelve days.

- After the skin glue comes off, you can begin wearing Steri-Strips™

on the suture line at all times for the six weeks following the removal of the sutures. These are provided by your surgeon.

- Avoid strenuous activity/lifting for at least three to four weeks post-op to prevent stretching of the incision. You may shower or bathe with the strips in place. However, you should change them periodically—remove them every five to seven days, bathe, dry the area gently, and then reapply.

WEEK SIX TO SIX MONTHS— MOISTURIZE/SOFTEN/PROTECT THE SKIN INCISIONS

- Begin using a moisturizing and hydrating cream twice daily by gently massaging it into the incision with a circular motion for six months. The key is to have an oil-free moisturizer and skin hydrator so you can enhance normal wound healing.

- The use of silicone gel is not warranted unless you are having a wound healing problem such as prolonged reddened appearance or an elevated scar.

- Protect the incision from the sun and use extra sunscreen on the scar—if you don't, it will take longer for the color to fade and blend with the rest of your skin.

SIX TO TWELVE MONTHS—SCAR MANAGEMENT/PROTECTION/ USE OF SUNSCREENS LONG TERM

- It is normal for scars to take twelve months or longer to see the final result—they may be hard, red, and numb for a long time, especially if you have pigmented skin.

- The scar will be reevaluated at this time. Very infrequently, scar revision may be needed but will not be performed until at least twelve to fifteen months after surgery, to allow for maximal wound healing.

- Use sunscreen on your incisions for life to prevent prolonged redness and pigmentation changes.

As you may have noted, all of the procedures listed above require you to refrain from exercise and sexual activity because it can result in increased swelling and bruising. If you have incisions, avoid strenuous activity and heavy lifting for at least four to six weeks. In the grand scheme of things, this is not that long and you will be back to your old life in short order. During recovery, you should really just focus on your healing. You'll have time to get back into shape later.

You also want to avoid direct sunlight on the surgical site for the first year. Try to wear clothing that covers the area—this can also help hide scars until they refine and fade. Continue to use a sunscreen with an SPF of 30 or higher and both UVA and UVB protection forever—scars have a slightly elevated risk for skin cancer when subjected to excessive UV rays, so it is important to keep them protected. And really, you should be using sunscreen over your entire body anyway, so this shouldn't be a concern.

Five Key Points:

1. **Follow your surgeon's post-op instructions carefully.** This book is a general guide, but no substitute for proper, expert medical care. Your surgeon may have other things he wants you to do, but these are the basics of good, essential post-op care.

2. **Each type of procedure is different as is each individual patient.** Every patient heals differently, so do not worry if your recovery takes longer than most. You will get there!

3. **Do not smoke, have sex, or restart an exercise or other daily routines without first clearing the changes with your surgeon.**

4. **Take care of yourself mentally and physically. Watch for early signs of post-op depression.** Some is normal so recognize it and surround yourself with a positive support group and surgical companion.

5. **Proper wound care is an important part of recovery for any surgery. Follow your surgeon's advice carefully. Good scar care starts with good wound care and transitions into good skin care for life.**

Lifelong Maintenance
... And Some Final Thoughts

13

The overall goal of this book has been to help you—the consumer and patient—navigate the world of plastic surgery safely and effectively so that you can achieve the ultimate care and outcome. Our hope is that you will find this book useful as a reference and guide both now and in the future. We have prepared you for all of the common plastic surgery procedures as well as equipped you with the knowledge to care for yourself and your body throughout each stage of life. We hope that we have provided you with the tools to be the very best you can be, always, no matter your age, gender, or lifestyle. This is what we all want as patients and people—to be our own personal best, physically, mentally, and spiritually. At this point you should understand:

- ***The vital role of the Three Magic Questions.*** *They will not fail you in finding the right plastic surgeon for you.*

- ***The importance of selecting the right plastic surgeon*** *for YOU by using Dr. Rohrich's Ten Point Guide to Selecting a Great Surgeon. You will be confident that you can find a surgeon who is truly an expert in their field.* ***Once you're in the surgeon's office, remember to ask the THREE MAGIC QUESTIONS. By now, you may feel as if we have belabored this point, and probably we have—the fact is that choosing a great surgeon is absolutely crucial to both ensuring your safety and optimal surgical outcomes. Your surgeon is not just the person performing your procedure but is also your guide—choosing the right person will dictate the ease with which you are able to navigate the entire process.***

The surgeon is someone you should completely trust and respect. Select your plastic surgeon with the same care and diligence with which you would select your family doctor. Your plastic surgeon, like your family doctor, is someone with whom you will want to stay with for life—someone who will be there as you move through all stages of life from your teens to your golden years.

- **Being the best starts and ends with you!** *Your surgeon is your guide, but you are the one who must take and navigate the journey. Only you can choose how to live your life, and it is ultimately up to you to make informed choices and stick to them. Taking care of your looks and your health is a lifelong endeavor. It begins with starting a medical-grade skin care regimen in your teens and following through with it for life. Some of the best things you can do are just this simple—but only you can do them for yourself.*

- **Your body's needs will evolve as you age and your maintenance regimen must keep pace.** *In your late twenties and thirties, you may want to begin incorporating neuromodulators like Botox® and/or fillers into your skin care regimen. As you continue to age further, you may find that body contouring and facial rejuvenation are necessary to maintain your youthful look. Your plastic surgeon will be your guide here, offering advice on how to continue to look your best through the years.*

- **It is imperative to do your research when considering plastic surgery.** *This book has given you the basic background knowledge and the know-how to pick the right surgeon and procedures as well as providing answers to all of your surgical questions. Remember the Three E's: Experience, Expertise, and Exceptional Results = the* **Three Magic Questions**.

You must understand the ins and outs of the procedure you are considering; whether it is a facelift, rhinoplasty, breast enhancement, body contouring surgery, or any other procedure. *You now have all the information necessary for making informed consumer and patient choices. You need to know what you can and cannot do with plastic* *surgery. Be realistic and choose the top three concerns that you want corrected.*

- ***The difficulties and limitations of secondary and revision surgery call for a "true expert" in the field***. *You should understand the benefits and limitations of secondary surgery and the need for a surgeon who is a true expert in a particular procedure.*

- ***How to prepare for your consultation—remember the three major concerns by using the Mirror Test***, *and refer to the step-by-step instructions to prepare for consultation and our list of must-ask questions in Chapter 3.*

- ***The general recovery process for surgery and the specific aftercare instructions for your procedure***. *Remember the importance of a good surgery companion.*

In the previous chapters, we explained that your journey as a plastic surgery patient does not end in the operating room and is not over until you have completely recovered and achieved your results. The rest of this chapter is dedicated to providing you with the tools and the knowledge to maintain and navigate your beauty for the rest of your life, along with knowing how to maintain your surgical results along with your natural beauty. Some of the following advice is specific to plastic surgery, but much of it is simply the recipe for overall physical and mental health. Keep this information and review it regularly. Let it be your guide, whether you are currently considering a procedure or not.

There are four main aspects to consider when it comes to maintaining your results after surgery. These steps are simple and straightforward, but they do take lifelong dedication and commitment. You need to:

- Understand and practice complete skin care. Refer to Chapter 4 for details on maintaining great skin.

- Take the necessary steps to Maximize Your Natural Beauty and maintain the results from your cosmetic surgery.

- Maintain an optimal healthy diet—for life.

- Develop and adhere to a comprehensive, lifelong exercise program.

Maintaining Your New Face and Body—for Life

Patients who undergo facial rejuvenation can have amazing improvements in the way they look and feel. These patients, of course, want to know if their results will last. As we discussed in Chapter 6, the added volume and shaping of a facelift are long term, but you will continue to age after your procedure and maintenance will be necessary over time.

As a patient, there are five essential steps you can take to maximize the results of your facelift for as long as possible:

1. *Commit to employing a medical-grade skin care regimen, as outlined by Dr. Rohrich in Chapter 4. That means using cleansers and hydrators, exfoliators, pigment controllers, restorative agents like Retin-A®, and protective agents such as sunscreen consistently for the rest of your life.*

2. *Don't smoke! It will age you on both the inside and outside. Smoking will reduce your lifespan by at least ten years if you smoke for more than ten years.*

3. *Avoid excessive sun exposure, which causes skin cancer and ages you and your skin dramatically.*

4. *Maintain a healthy lifelong diet and exercise program that keeps your mind and body fit.*

5. Work with your plastic surgeon to maintain your results. You will continue to age even after having aesthetic plastic surgery—such is life. Do not be afraid to seek ancillary procedures to maintain your results as the years go by. You can supplement your primary

facial rejuvenation results with ongoing neuromodulators, fillers, and facial peels as needed. You may even find that, after many years, a secondary facelift may be in order.

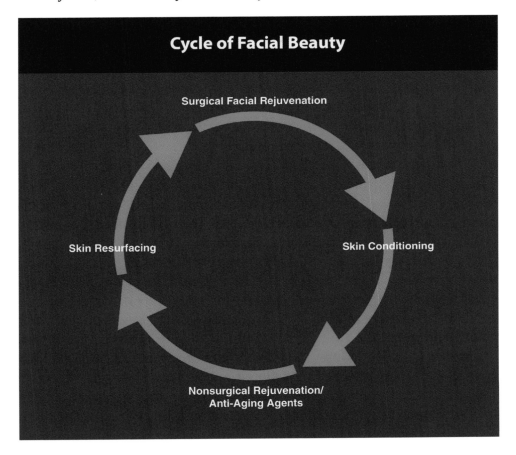

Cycle of Facial Beauty

Surgical Facial Rejuvenation

Skin Resurfacing

Skin Conditioning

Nonsurgical Rejuvenation/
Anti-Aging Agents

Non-surgical maintenance and preventative care are the best ways for patients to maintain their results. Surgical maintenance is no substitute for practicing due diligence when it comes to taking great care of your skin, face, and body. You will never be able to use surgery to counteract bad lifestyle habits and poor skin care. Taking good care of your body will actually minimize the need for further surgery, which is ideal. You cannot stop aging, but you can certainly continue to roll back the clock or slow it down by doing all of the above.

You do not need to continually return for surgery. Most patients can simply do ongoing maintenance where necessary to compensate for continued aging. The face tends to age more noticeably and rapidly than any other part of the body. The indications for a secondary facelift or fill are the same as when you were considering your primary facelift procedure: sagging skin and loss of volume. Generally speaking, a good facelift lasts approximately ten years on average. In practice, I am often able to extend that time period from ten to fifteen years with regular maintenance. You shouldn't need or consider a secondary facelift until after this amount of time *if* you follow our regular maintenance protocols.

Nutrition and Exercise—The Key to Maintaining Your Youthful Figure (and Your Surgical Results!)

Proper nutrition and exercise are equally important to maintaining your surgery results and your overall health. Living a healthy lifestyle and maintaining your weight are largely dependent upon proper nutrition. Exercise is important, but the quality and quantity of the foods that you put into your mouth are the leading factors in maintaining good health and, by extension, the youthful look and feel you achieved through surgery.

Let's focus on diet. Note that I mean "diet" and not "a diet." The word diet tends to invoke thoughts of short-term, on-again-off-again food restrictions—diet as a restrictive meal plan. This idea was popularized during the twentieth century through fad diets. Calorie restriction programs will only help you achieve transient weight loss at best. **The vast majority of people put the weight back on very quickly. That is because "a diet" is a short-term correction rather than an ongoing lifestyle change. These diets are impossible to maintain because most aren't designed with permanence in mind.** They intentionally leave you hungry while on them, and the weight usually comes right back once you go off.

That's what "a diet" is. But when we say "diet," we mean the types of foods that one normally consumes over one's lifetime. Think of your diet as your overall nutritional intake. Your diet is your food lifestyle. This kind of diet is much easier to maintain because, rather than focusing only on what you cannot eat, it focuses on what you can eat as well.

To help you make the right decisions, we have compiled a list of guidelines to facilitate appropriate choices about food and nutrition.

- **You are what you eat. There is more than a grain of truth to this old cliché. Food is literally what you put into your body and contains the fuel and building blocks with which your cells regenerate and reform. What we put into our bodies is what we are and dictates how we look and feel.**

  If you are constantly eating food that is high in calories, very processed, and loaded with salt, preservatives, and unnatural ingredients, you will probably battle weight gain throughout your life. Try to avoid processed foods and most foods in a box that have a shelf life (prepared whole foods don't usually last months or years!). This doesn't mean that you can never have those types of foods. But it does mean they can't comprise a significant portion of your regular diet. A slice of cake is not going to ruin your life, but a slice of cake a day, or perhaps every week, may affect the way you look and feel. You need to practice moderation—another bit of clichéd advice that, unfortunately, just happens to be true.

- **Consume foods from all of the major food groups**. We are not talking about the dated FDA "Food Pyramid" that probably had you eating way too many processed grains as a child.

  The three major food groups are:

  - **Proteins:** These are crucial for maintaining proper cellular growth and body function. I recommend a high protein diet, especially when recovering from surgery, as your body needs protein to create new cells (which is why it is also important for skin care). Good sources of protein are chicken, fish, and lean meats. I advise limiting red meat to lean cuts once or twice per week. Vegetarian sources of protein include quinoa, beans, and tofu, just to name a few.

  - **Carbohydrates:** These have been much maligned in recent years, but they are required for energy production and are absolutely necessary to good health. However, the average

American eats far too many carbohydrates and the wrong ones. **Not all carbs are created equal.** Stay away from simple carbohydrates that digest rapidly and cause spikes in insulin, which can lead to weight gain and diabetes. Candy, cakes, processed snack foods, and breads are just a few examples of simple carbohydrates and should be avoided. You should be getting most of your carbohydrates from nutrient-packed fresh fruits and vegetables.

- **Fats:** Another much maligned but absolutely necessary food group. Just as with carbohydrates, there are healthy fats and unhealthy fats. The key is to focus on consuming unsaturated fats while avoiding saturated fats and trans fats. Some foods naturally high in healthy unsaturated fats include avocados, salmon, olive oil, and flax seeds. **Scientific studies have shown that foods containing these good fats will actually lower your total cholesterol levels and increase healthy HDL cholesterol, which decreases your risk for heart disease.**

- **Know which foods YOU should avoid.** You don't have to have a full-blown food allergy to develop a food intolerance. Consider minimizing your consumption of foods containing gluten, such as wheat and barley. Gluten has been shown to cause inflammation in the digestive track, and more and more Americans are becoming gluten intolerant or allergic due to heredity or overexposure. You may also find that you are intolerant of lactose (found in dairy products) or other foods.

Food intolerances are specific to individuals! What bothers another person may not bother you, and vice versa. Consider an elimination diet and pay close attention to how you feel as you reintroduce foods. Anything that makes you feel tired or nauseated should be avoided. This is very common. I cannot eat a lot of carbs that are wheat-based like pasta and bread without feeling tired and sometimes ill. Listen to your body and it will tell you what it can't tolerate.

- **Stay hydrated.** Water is essential for life. The human body is composed of 70 percent water. We must replace water that our bodies lose through sweating, urination, and breathing. Luckily, your body has its own dehydration alert system—thirst. The problem is that many people have become so accustomed to chronic dehydration that they may miss or ignore the signs of dehydration, including being thirsty. So it can be good to think about water intake, especially if you are trying to take care of your skin, which needs adequate moisture to stay healthy. I advise my patients to consume three liters of water per day. You get on average one liter of water a day from food, which means you should drink two liters a day, which equates to approximately eight 8-ounce glasses of water per day. Adjust your intake for ambient temperature, activity level, and the moisture-content of your food intake. On exercise days you should drink an extra liter, or four more glasses of water.

  Drinking large amounts of water without eating can throw off your electrolyte balance, which can cause cramping. Even if you have never experienced painful or debilitating cramping, your body still needs a consistent and adequate supply of electrolytes in order to maintain all bodily functions at optimal levels. Cramping, like thirst, is your body's way of signaling that something is not right. Do not wait until your body is cramping or thirsty to replenish water and electrolytes, and you will be able to keep your body performing smoothly without interruption or compromise. You don't wait for your car's engine to start breaking down before getting an oil change, do you? Thirst means you are already dehydrated and cramping means you are already electrolyte deficient. Consistent replenishment of electrolytes is just as important as the food you consume and the water you drink during exercise. You can replenish your electrolytes easily through proper diet or with enhanced electrolytes drinks if you are exercising. Avoid *carbonated drinks and sodas. They cause bloating and also deplete your body of certain nutrients, such as calcium and magnesium, which are important to your immune system.*

- **Portion control is everything.** Even healthy foods aren't healthy when overeaten. If you think your portions might be too large, they probably are. Restaurants have trained us to expect larger portions. Too much food usually means too many calories. Reasonable portions also allow you to eat small meals throughout the day, which helps prevent your blood sugar from fluctuating. It is important to know what a portion size looks like. Your portions of protein should be about the size of a deck of cards or the size of your palm (not both palms combined)—so you need to start cutting those sixteen-ounce steaks into quarters! Vegetables and fruit portions should be about a half cup of each, or about the size of a baseball.

  A hamburger loaded down with cheese and condiments and served with fries can easily have in excess of one or two thousand calories. Think about that—that's just one meal! It's not hard to see how one can put weight on so quickly. You need to watch your portion control and your daily intake to take control of your weight.

- **Remain aware of your caloric intake and expenditure.** Calories are a measure of the energy we get from food. Excess calories are stored as fat by the body, and putting on excess fat is obviously not conducive to maintaining surgery outcomes. Our optimal daily caloric need varies based on gender, age, and physical activity. For example, a moderately active forty-year-old man may only need approximately 2,500 calories per day, whereas a moderately active forty-year-old woman's needs should range from approximately 1,700–1,800 calories per day. These numbers are examples approximate for maintenance only—if you need to lose weight, you may need to restrict your daily caloric intake by about 500 calories. Speak with a nutritionist about your caloric needs and how to balance your intake with your energy expenditure.

  While portion control is key to taking control of your "calories in versus calories out" balance, it's important not to deprive your body of food—this can actually slow your metabolism, paradoxically causing you to gain weight. Remember to think of diet as a lifestyle and you will have an easier time maintaining it day in and day out.

- **Watch your sodium intake.** Sodium is a necessary nutrient and electrolyte, but we consume far too much. The average American consumes 6000 to 8000 grams of sodium a day even though the recommended guidelines are less than 2300 milligrams per day or less than 1500 milligrams for those over fifty. These limits are probably even too high. The human body really *needs only about 500 milligrams* of sodium each day, perhaps up to 2000 milligrams if you are an athlete. You can get this amount simply by eating natural, unprocessed foods. Sodium occurs naturally in whole foods. Too much sodium contributes to heart disease, congestive heart failure, stroke, and chronic kidney disease. It also causes bloating, which will make you appear heavier than you actually are.

- **Vitamins are necessary, but that doesn't necessarily mean you need to take packaged vitamins.** All of the vitamins you need can be derived from the foods you eat. In fact, they are best absorbed by the body this way. If you make good food choices and eat a variety of healthy foods from all food groups, you are probably already getting all of the vitamins your body needs. If you are concerned or have reason to believe you are vitamin deficient, you can have a blood panel done to check for deficiencies.

Yes, You Have to Exercise

No matter how good your diet is, you still need to exercise for optimal health. Simply put: you need not make this complicated. Adopt a simple exercise program that you adhere to consistently. You should try to work out a minimum five days per week—daily is even better. You can find lifelong success with many different types of exercise programs. Maybe you want to try yoga. Perhaps you prefer the all-in approach of CrossFit®. Some prefer the camaraderie of team sports while others prefer solo activities, such as biking or running. Your exercise routine should include both cardiovascular training and light weight training (which can also be body weight only). You do not have to do both every day—you can rotate between cardio and weight training on alternate days.

When it comes to cardio, you want to do either 150 minutes of moderate aerobic exercise or 75 minutes of vigorous aerobic exercise per week. We define vigorous exercise as anything that gets you to 70 to 80 percent of your maximum heart rate. How do you estimate your maximum heart rate?

Here is one of the simple formulas you can use. Simply subtract your age from 220 and then multiply by .70 or 70%, and this will give the heart rate to reach. For example, a woman who is forty-five years old would use the following (220–45 = 175 x .70 = 122). For 80% do the same (220–45 = 175 x .80 = 140). So she would want to have her heart rate somewhere between 122–140 beats per minute while vigorously exercising.

Congratulations—at this point, you should understand the basics of proper diet and exercise! The key is to find a healthy exercise routine that fits into your lifestyle, one that you can and will adhere to over the long term, and to be acutely aware of the foods you are putting into your body and their effects upon you. If it seems simple, that's because it is! The above diet and exercise plan is meant to make choosing a healthy lifestyle as simple and straightforward as possible.

But What if I Need to Lose Weight?

The diet and exercise guidelines apply to those who are looking to maintain their weight. If you are interested in losing weight, you may need to make a few slight alterations until you hit your target weight:

- **Exercise longer and talk to a professional.** You may need to increase your weekly cardio routine to approximately 250 minutes per week (approximately 30–35 minutes per day). This will help.

- **Vigorous exercise will get you burning calories faster.** Your goal should be to reach and maintain 70 percent of your maximum heart rate as soon as possible. Vigorous exercise may leave you out of breath (though not to where you cannot talk) but will certainly jump-start weight loss. Not everyone is in good enough physical health to start out exercising so vigorously and you do not want to injure yourself. Listen to your body and work your way up. For weight training, you can start by simply using your own body weight, performing light exercises such as push-ups, squats, and lunges. You then may want to advance to using weight resistance, such as resistance bands, free weights, or weight machines. If sprinting and distance running are too difficult at first, you can start doing cardio exercises by simply walking at a fast pace, light jogging, or bike riding. Whatever you do, aim for at least 30 minutes five to six times per week and work your way up.

- **Reduce calories.** Remember your caloric intake versus outtake balance. To lose weight, you will need to reduce your maximum calorie allowance based on your age, weight, gender, and activity level.

- **Do not eat before bed.** Your metabolism goes way down while you sleep, and those nighttime calories have a way of converting to fat. Avoid food for at least three hours before bedtime.

- **You may want to consider hiring a personal trainer to help you stay on track.** This can really help if you tend to put off exercise and weight loss. A good trainer will also keep you accountable.

- **You may want to consider body contouring.** If you are within 10 to 15 pounds of your ideal weight but cannot seem to drop the last few pounds in resistant areas of the body, such as around the waist, hips, or thighs, you may be a prime candidate for liposuction and/or body contouring that will restore a trim and youthful figure that matches your already healthy lifestyle. But realize that liposuction absolutely cannot be used to remove massive amounts of weight. Refer back to Chapter 9 for more on liposuction and body contouring.

- **Savor your food.** Eat and chew your food slowly. When you are eating, focus on your meal, not the television or other distractions that can lead to mindless eating and overeating. Serve yourself a moderately sized portion and resist the temptation to go back for seconds.

- **Understand that food is a powerful drug that affects the way our bodies function.** High-fat and—especially—high-carb foods can be addictive. Two-thirds of the American population is obese because we are literally addicted to destructive processed foods. But you don't have to be—become aware of what you eat, don't abuse your body, and be the best you can be. That's what good health and aesthetic surgery are all about.

These are only recommendations. You may find that simply following the above guidelines for leading a healthy lifestyle may be enough to bring you down to your target weight, but some people need to put in a little extra effort due to physiological idiosyncrasies. Everyone is different—find what works for you and also realize that what works for you will change over time. I am still making regular adjustments to my diet and exercise routines and it works! And if it doesn't, I change it up.

Final Thoughts

As we stated at the outset, my co-author, Mary Crosland, and I wrote this book to teach you to better navigate your life for both your inner and outer beauty. We hope that you have found these health and beauty principles to be helpful and even, perhaps, life changing. As you begin your journey towards looking and feeling the best you can, we hope this book serves as your guide. **We want to help you be the best "you" that you can be.**

This book will help you receive the best and safest care possible. Knowing how to choose the right surgeon will help you make decisions ranging from skin care, fillers, facial rejuvenation, breast enhancement, body contouring, revision and secondary surgery, or other plastic surgery procedures.

You are now an informed consumer and know how to find a true expert in plastic surgery. You can NAVIGATE YOUR BEAUTY with smart and safe plastic surgery solutions designed with you in mind.

Good luck . . . and let us know what procedure you choose, how you select your surgeon, and what results you get. We want to hear from you as you begin to navigate your beauty for life on **navigateyourbeauty.com!**